MEDICINAL PLANTS

Donated to your Library by the author,

Unedosa

4/3/2023

UCHECHUKWU A. UTOH-NEDOSA, PHD,

Lecturer (Rtd), Department of Pharmacology and Toxicology, Faculty of Pharmaceutical Sciences, Nnamdi Azikiwe University, Awka, Nigeria, West Africa, Africa

Fulton Books, Inc.
Meadville, PA

Published by Fulton Books 2021

ISBN 978-1-63710-417-0 (paperback)
ISBN 978-1-63710-418-7 (digital)

Printed in the United States of America

CONTENTS

ACKNOWLEDGMENTS

WISH TO USE this opportunity to thank Almighty God for providing medicinal plants to heal diseases and health disorders of humans, animals, and fellow plants.

INTRODUCTION

KNOWLEDGE OF MEDICINAL plants is essential for understanding and use of complementary and alternative medicine.

This book gives many examples of medicinal plants, describes the medicinal effects of these plants, and describes their mechanisms of action in the body.

This book will be informative to many people in the world who currently want to include more plant-based foods and "herbs" in their diets. It will also educate those people who want to take plant materials as infusions/effusions or as smoothies to obtain micronutrients.

There are pharmacological and physiological effects of medicinal plant extracts in the body.

WHO WILL BENEFIT FROM THIS BOOK?

THIS BOOK WILL be benefitted from by every member of the general public of all ages, as the book enables everyone to know many medicinal plants and the family of plants they belong to, in order to better use medicinal plants as food or to produce micronutrients needed by the body for health promotion. The book will be of immense benefit to college and university students and students of other tertiary institutions especially students of nutrition, dietetics, food science, physical and natural sciences, medical and paramedical sciences, pharmaceutical and agricultural sciences, traditional and herbal medicine, etc. Scientific facts about the medicinal effects produced in the body by a large number of medicinal plants which can be used for food or for production of alternative medicines, to promote health or as adjunct therapy, are in this book. The book also helps readers to better understand the effects of medicinal herbs or plant materials they are already using as food or food condiment or as alternative medicines. The book also uses scientific research studies on medicinal plants to teach the scientific basis of claims that those plants produce medicinal effects in the body.

CHAPTER 1

What Are Medicinal Plants?

MILLIONS OF TREES all over the world have medicinal effects. Only a fraction of them has been identified and employed for medicinal purposes by humans. This book describes many medicinal plants, their extracts, and their juices. The book also describes the medicinal effects of medicinal plants that have been identified through scientific studies done with the extracts and juices of various parts of medicinal plants

Medicinal plants are, first and foremost, "plants," after which they are "medicinal." This means that medicinal plants perform other functions that plants perform for humans. Also, when they are taken into the body, they produce some pharmacological effects that affect the body's physiology. The chemical constituents of extracts of medicinal plants are designed to "know" or recognize what the normal body physiology is and to recognize when the body's physiology is deranged by disease or health disorder. Hence, when inhibitory plant extracts or juices reach a deranged site of the body or notice a deranged body's physiological function, they correct the disordered state of the body.

Green plants use carbon dioxide of the atmosphere for the manufacture of their own food. Carbon dioxide combines with the chlorophyll (the green coloring matter of plants present in the chloroplast of their cells), in the presence of sunlight (as their source of energy) to produce their own food (carbohydrates) and release oxygen into the atmosphere. Photosynthesizing medicinal plants also manufacture and store excess foods they produce for use of humans. Medicinal plants also provide wood, gum, resin, and other bye-product of plants.

Medicinal plants have constituents that produce health-promoting or health-healing effects on the body cells or organs of humans, animals, and themselves or other plants. Medicinal plants can be found near homes, in farms, in grasslands, in bushes, in forests, and in wet or arid zones of the earth. The ubiquity of medicinal plants is probably next to that of air and water on the earth's surface.

Even remains of dead plants, some of which died in ages past, have been found to have medicinal effects. In Nigeria, for example, petroleum crude oil, which resulted from compressed remains of plants that died in ages past, is used as folk medicine for the treatment of arthritic and many ill-health conditions. Pith derived from compressed masses of dead moss is officially used in the pharmaceutical industry to make wound dressing while dead Iceland moss is used for the treatment of gastrointestinal disorders. Many medicinal plants are used as their dried leaves, stems, stem bark, root, root bark, flowers, fruits, fruit rinds, seeds, et cetera. Thus, even after death, the remains of medicinal plants continue to provide medicines for the cure of ailments of living organisms.

Some medicinal plants whose drugs have been in use for years in orthodox medicine and as research tools include *Cinchona* of family *Rubiaceae* from which the antimalarial quinine was produced and ipecac of the plant *Cephaelis ipecacuana* (family *Rubiaceae*) from which emetine used for the treatment of intestinal amoebiasis and sheep liver fluke infestation was produced. Other examples of orthodox drugs derived from medicinal plants include pilocarpine (which is derived from the leaves of *Pilocarpus jaborandi*) used in ophthalmology as a miotic and for stimulating the flow of saliva in patients who complain of the dryness of mouth during therapy with ganglion blocking agents; belladonna alkaloids, atropine (l-hyoscine), and scopolamine (l-hyoscine) from the solanaceous plant called the deadly nightshade and *Atropa belladonna*; and hyoscyamine derived from henbane (*Hyoscamus niger*), which find uses in ophthalmology, anesthesia, and in cardiac and gastrointestinal disease treatment. Others still are physostigmine or eserine, an antidote in atropine poisoning derived from the Calabar or ordeal bean; reserpine, with antihypertensive and tranquilizing properties derived from *Rauwolfia serpentina* alkaloids; d-tubocurarine (the active principle of the roots of *Chondodendron tomentosu*), a competitive neuromuscular blocking agent which produces flaccid paralysis of the extremities, employed in anesthesiology; and strychnine (a complex alkaloid obtained from the seeds of the plant *Strychnos nux vomica*), which exerts a predominant effect on the spinal cord, that lowers the threshold of excitability of various neurons so that any sudden stimulation of the animal (such as stimulation with noise), precipitates a tonic extensor seizure.

Other plant-derived orthodox drugs that are also more well-known are morphine and codeine employed in relief of severe pain, and papaverine (whose main pharmacologic effect is smooth muscle relaxation and a moderate quinidine-like effect on the heart). Papaverine is obtained from the plant *Paperver somniferum*, which is used in folk medicine as an analgesic and a soporific.

The chemical constituents of many aromatic and pungent plant spices and condiments used for food and beverage flavoring and seasoning have medicinal properties. Examples of these aromatic spices include ginger, *Zingiber officinale* (family Zingiberaceae); cardamoms (*Elettaria cardamomum* [family Zingiberaceae]); black pepper (*Piper nigrum* [family Piperaceae]); red or chili pepper (*Capsicum annum* [family *Solanaceae*]); cloves (*Syzygium aromaticum* [family Myrtaceae]); garlic (*Allium sativum* [family Liliaceae]); onions (*Allium cepa* [family Liliaceae]); cinnamon (*Cinnamomum zeynalicum* [family *Lauraceae*]); bay leaf (*Cinnam omum tamala* [family Lauraceae]); and Ethiopian pepper (*Xylopia aethiopica* [family *Annonaceae*]), just to name a few.

Many plants serve multiple economic uses. Thus, some plants or plant products that serve as food, beverages, vegetables, desserts, edible and industrial oils, spices and food/beverage condiments, timber-producing trees, fiber-producing trees, paper mills' raw-material producers, etc.; also produce medicinal products. The following food plants, for example, also produce folk medicinal products: maize (*Zea mays* [family Gramminae]), sweet potatoes (*Ipomea digitate* and *Ipomea batatas* [family Convolvulaceae]), yams (*Dioscorea* spp. [family Dioscoreaceae]), cassava (*Manihot esculentus* [family Euphorbiaceae]), and soya beans (*Glycine max*). The following fruits that are also used for foods, salads, or desserts yield medicinal products: pawpaw (*Carica papaya* [family *Caricaceae*]), mango (*Magifera indica* [family *Anacardiaceae*]), orange (*Citrus reticulata* [family Rutacea]), pineapple (*Ananas cosmosus* [family Bromeliaceae]), and banana (*Musa paradisiaca* [family Musaceae]), just to name a few.

Many spices and beverage condiments also yield medicinal products. Their examples include some that have been mentioned above like cloves, pepper, cinnamon, ginger, and *Xylopia* species. Some others are chamomile (pomegranate fusion), cocoa (*Theobroma cacao* [family *Sterculiaceae*]), coffee (*Coffea arabica* and *Coffea robusta* [family Rubiaceae]), and tea (*Tea assamica* and *Thea sienensis* [family Theaceae]).

Timber-producing plants that can also yield medicinal products include Indian redwood (*Dalbergia sissoo* [family Paplionaceae]), mahogany (*Swietenia mahagoni* [family Meliaceae]) and pines (*Pinus longifolia* and *Pinus khasya* [family Abietaceae]).

Fiber-producing plants that can also yield medicinal products include jute (*Corchorus capsularis* and *Corchorus olitorius* [family *Tiliaceae*]), cotton (*Gossypium* spp. [family Malvaceae]) and hemp (*Cannabis sativa* [family Cannabinaceae]).

The plant *Hevea brasilensis* (family Euphorbiaceae) is the main source of commercial rubber that is used for the making of tubes and tires; insulation of electrical wires; rubber soles of shoes; and for minor use as gum material. Gum arabic tree yields gum as well as some folk medicinal products.

Some oilseeds and fruits also produce folk medicinal products. Examples of these include sesame seed, mustard seed, groundnut seed, sunflower seed, star anise seed, *Theobroma* spp. seed, soya beans, castor oil seed, *Borago officinalis* seed and palm kernel seed.

Some Practical Examples of Medicinal Plants

Among the Igbos of Southeastern Nigeria, medicinal plants that can also serve for food or other economic uses are planted within and immediately outside the external compound walls. A few samples of these medicinal plants used in Igbo folk medicine found inside and outside the compound walls are shown in the photographic plates below.

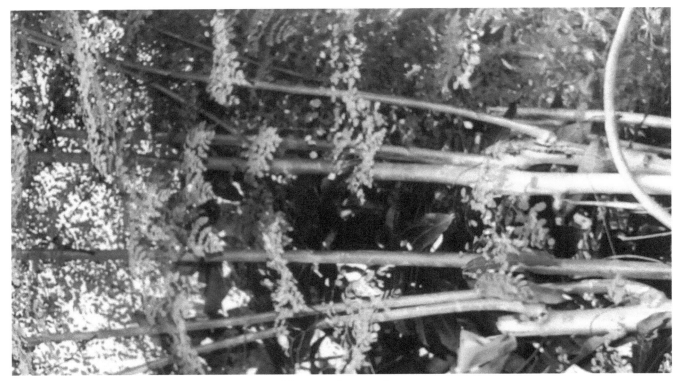

Moringa oleovera plant

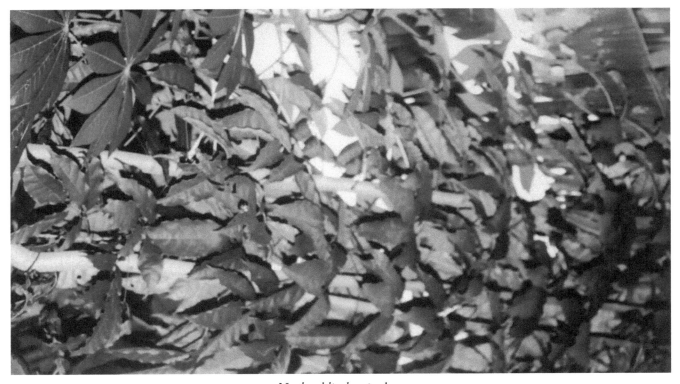

Neubouldia laevis plant

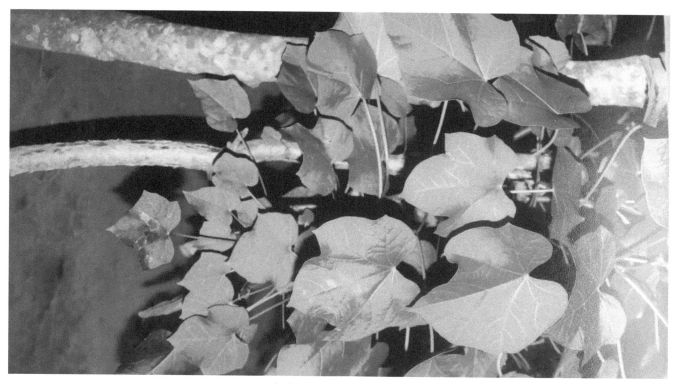

Ugbokoro (Igbo name) plant

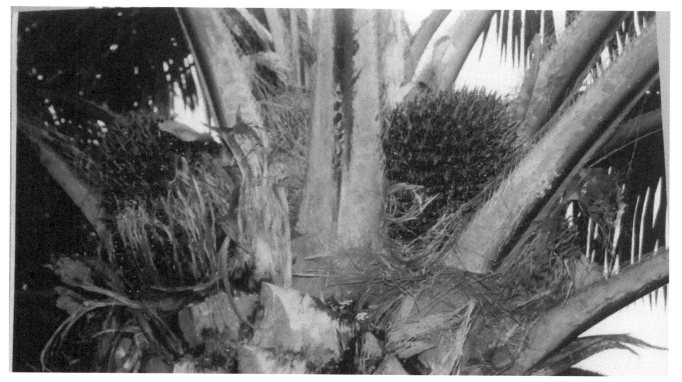

The tip of an oil palm tree

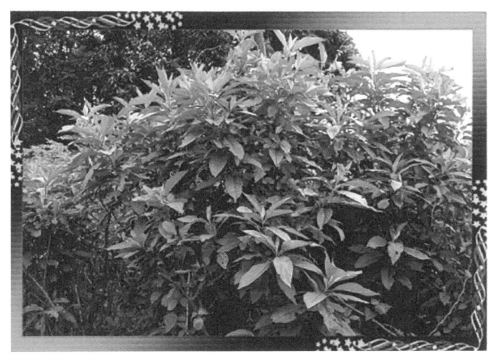

Vernonia amygdalina (bitter leaf) shrub

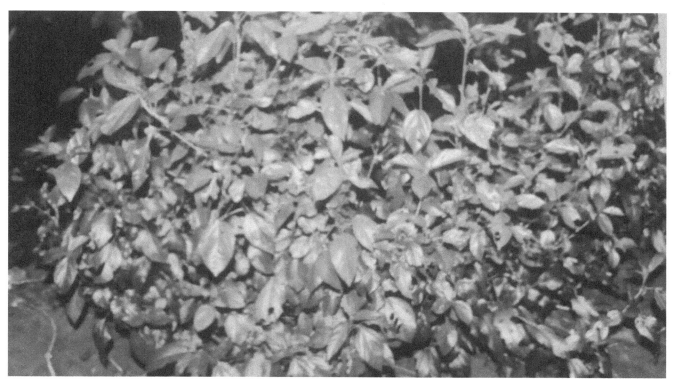

Ahihaa (Igbo name) plant, a vegetable that produces gumlike extract in water that is usually more "sticky" or gummy than that produced by cut soft okra fruits

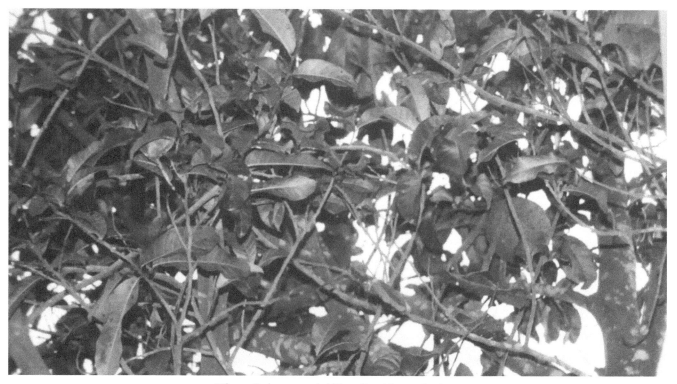

Ukwa (Igbo name) (*Treculia Africana*) plant

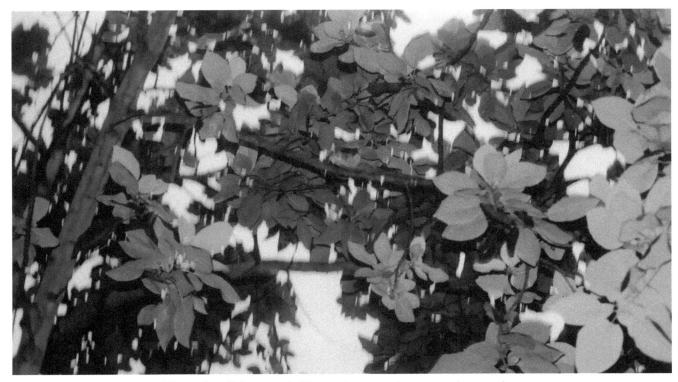

Ube oyibo (Igbo name) (*Persea Americana*) or avocado pea plant

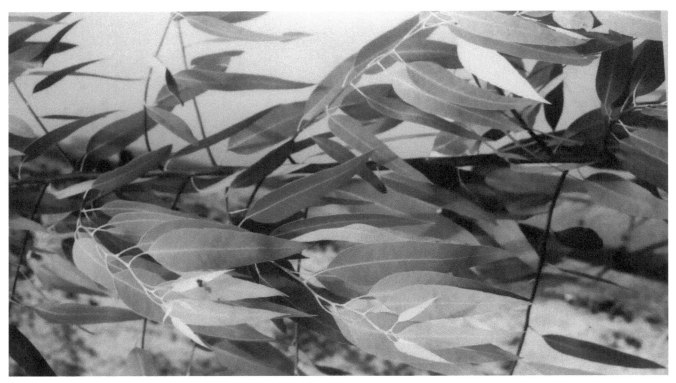

Eucalyptus spp. plant

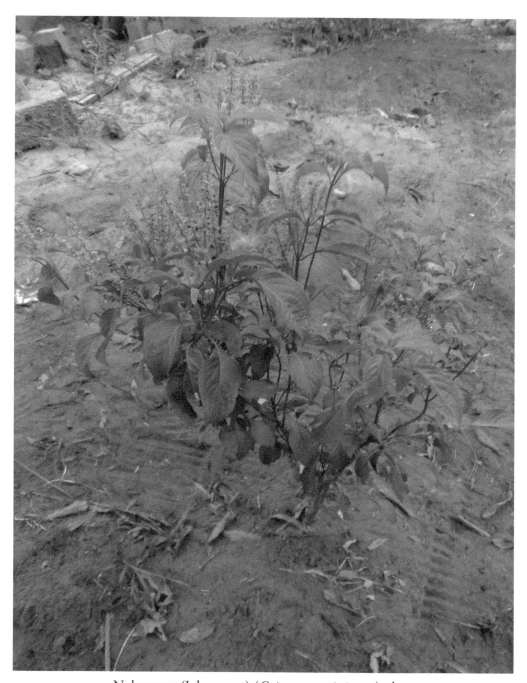

Ngbuanwu (Igbo name) (*Ocimum gratissimum*) plant

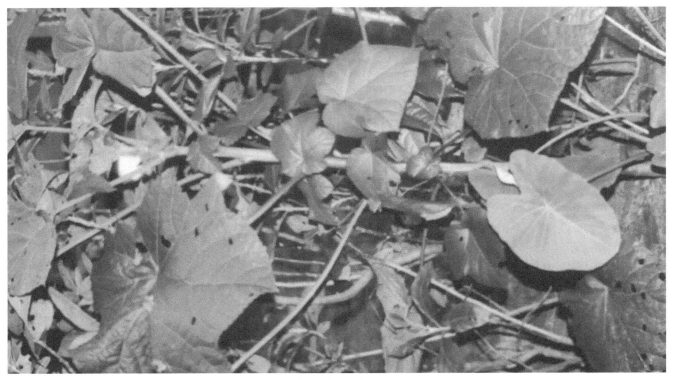

Okra plant (*front*)

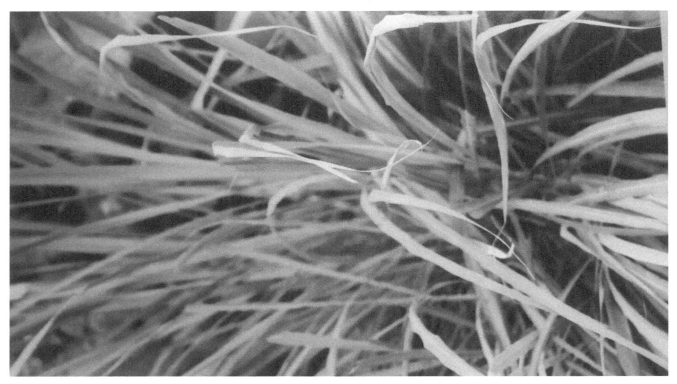

Lemongrass (*Cymbopogon citratus*) plant

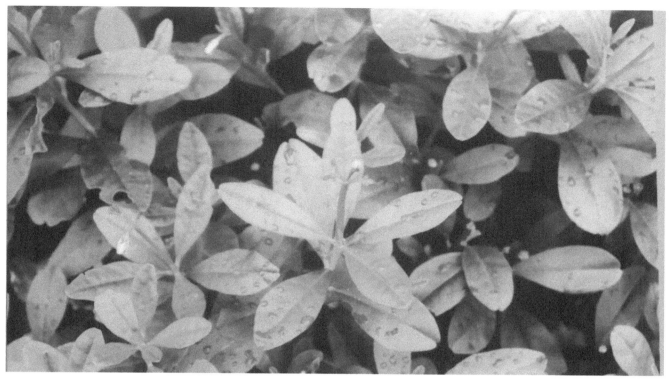

Waterleaf or Gborongi (Igbo name) (*Talinum triangulare*) plant

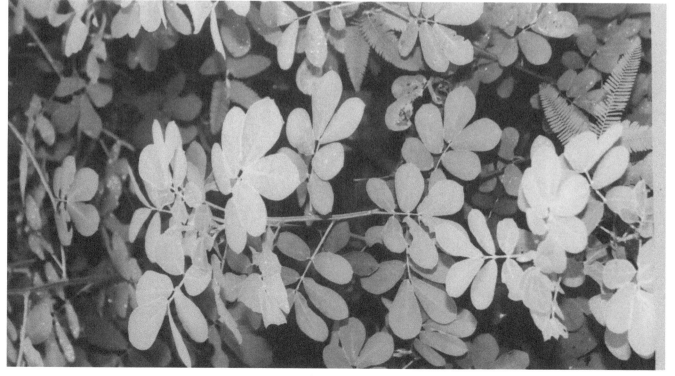

Caesalpina spp. plant

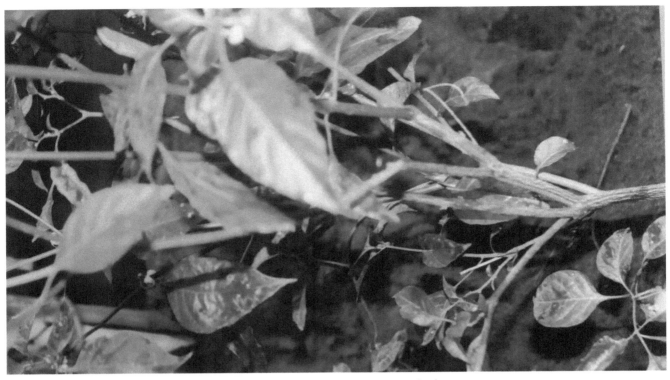

Ose (Igbo name) (*Capsicum annum*) plant

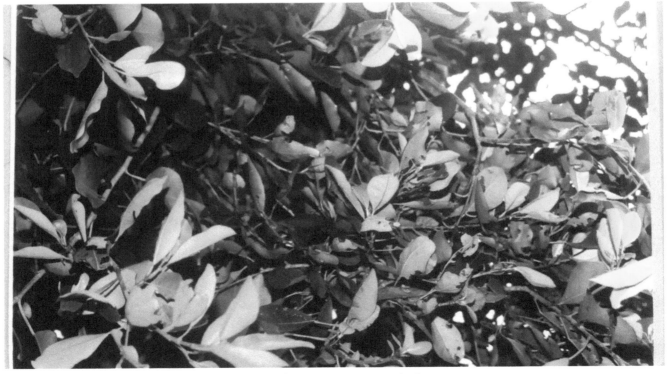

Ogbu (Igbo name) (*Ficus* spp.) plant

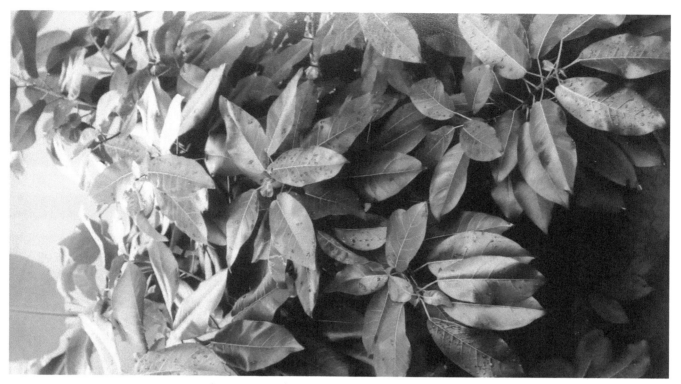

Another species of *Ficus* spp. (Ogbu) (Igbo name) plant

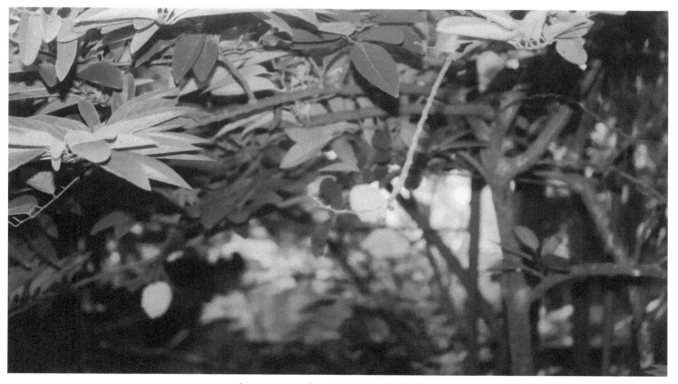

Annona spp. (sweetsop species) plant

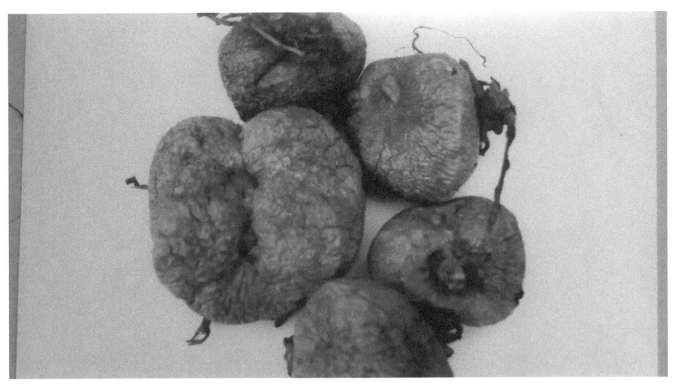

Adu (Igbo name) or "bitter" yam (yam that has a bitter taste). Adu is no longer widely planted.

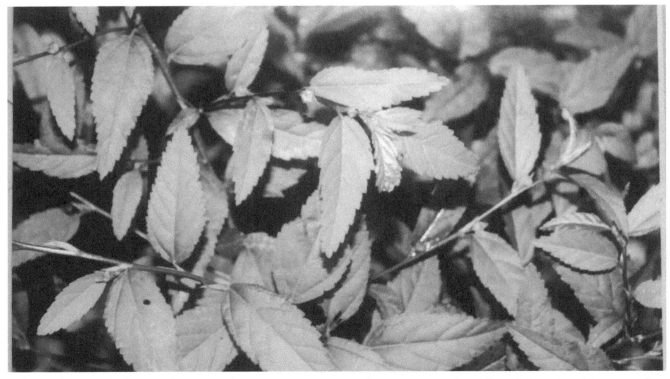

Udoo (Igbo name) plant. Its leaves produce gummy extract, and its stem is used as a "rope" for tying things together.

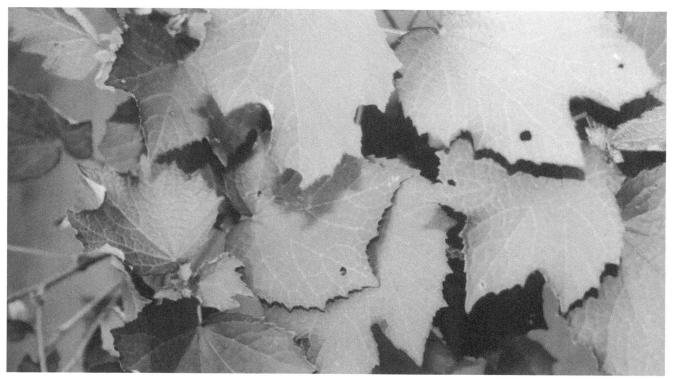

Another species of Udoo also produces gummy liquid extract like aloe vera. Its stem is also used as a "rope" for tying bundles of things like wood.

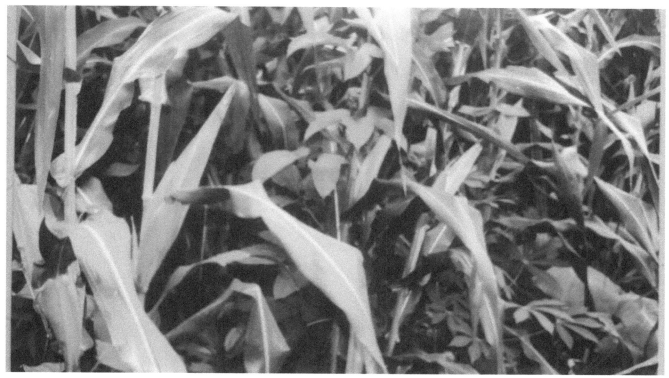

Oka (Igbo name) (*Zea mays*) or maize plant.

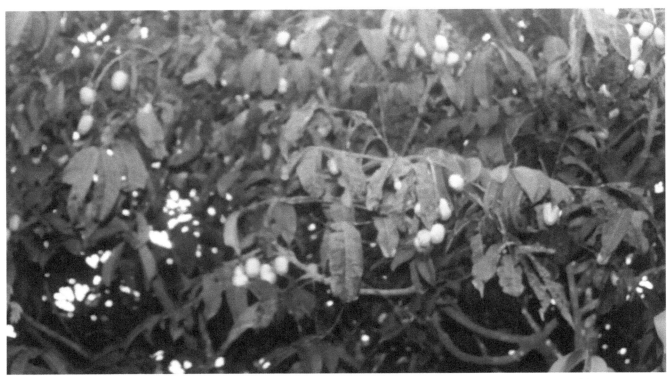

Ube (Igbo name) tree, an indigenous pea tree. The bark of these indigenous pea trees yields strong gum that resembles but is stronger than the gum of gum arabica trees.

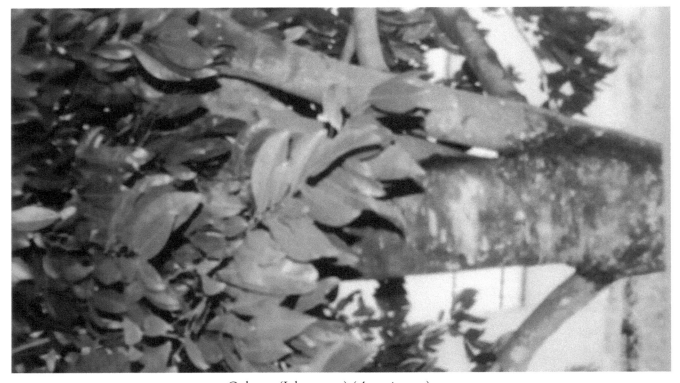

Ogbono (Igbo name) (*Avengia* spp.) tree

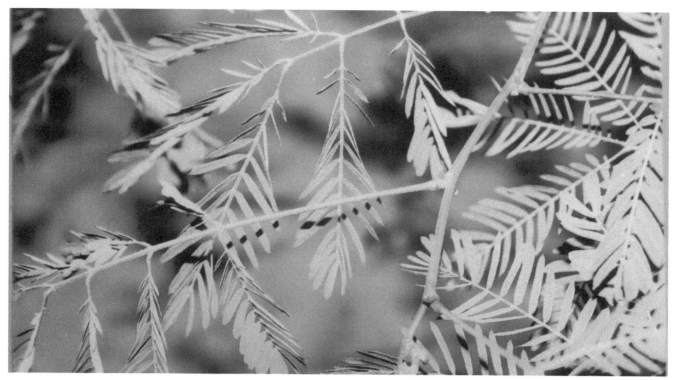

Mimosa spp. tree

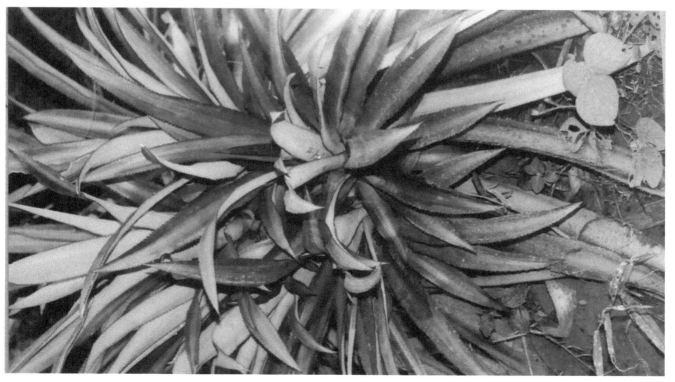

Oka Nkwu (Igbo name) or pineapple plant

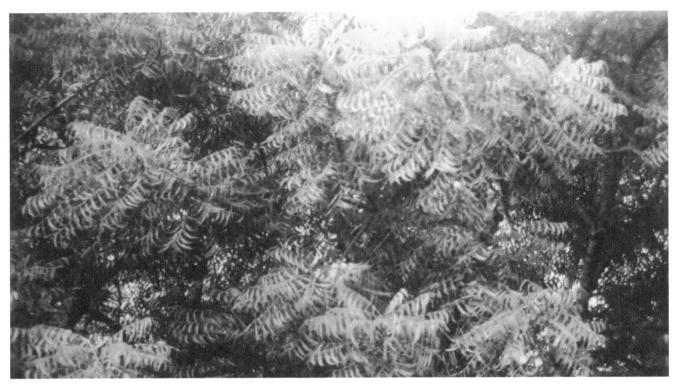

Dogon Yaro (Hausa name) or Neem tree (*Azadirachta indica*)

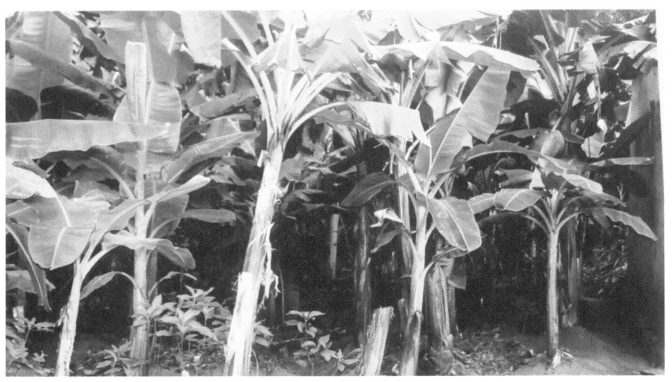

Ojoko or Ji Okoh (Igbo name) (*Musa* spp. [plantain giant herbs])

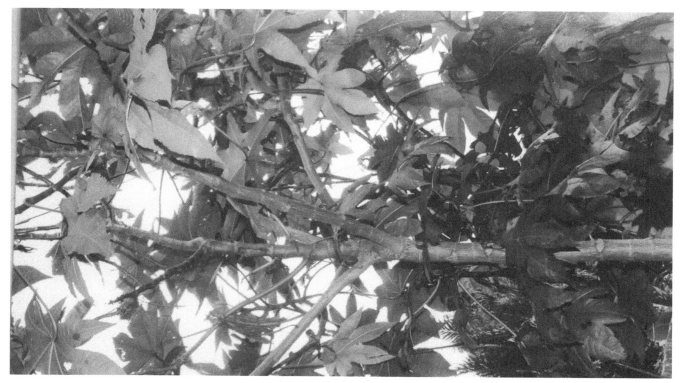

Ogiri Ugba (Igbo name) (*Ricinis communis*)

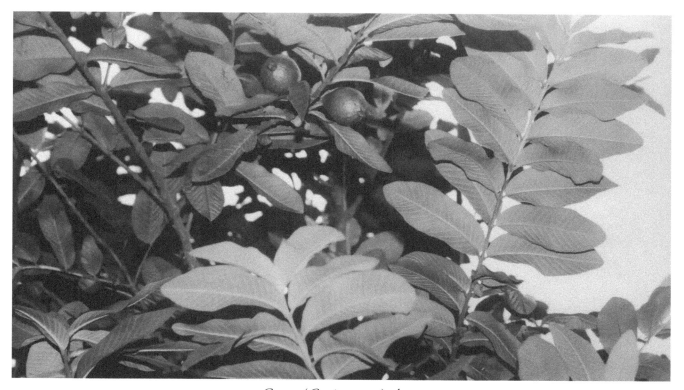

Guava (*Guajava* spp.) plant

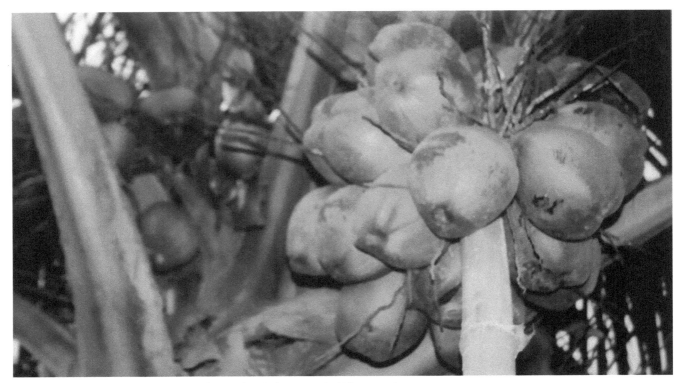

Aki Oyibo (Igbo name) (*Eleis cocoa*) or coconut tree

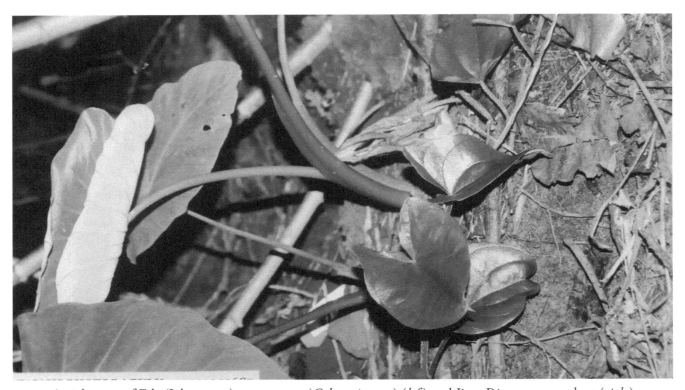

Aerial stems of Ede (Igbo name) or cocoyam (*Colocassia* spp.) (*left*) and Ji or *Dioscorea* spp. plant (*right*)

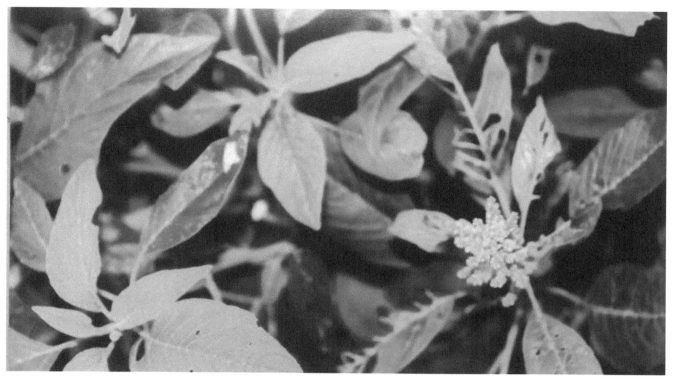

Amaranthus spp. or Inine (Igbo name) plant

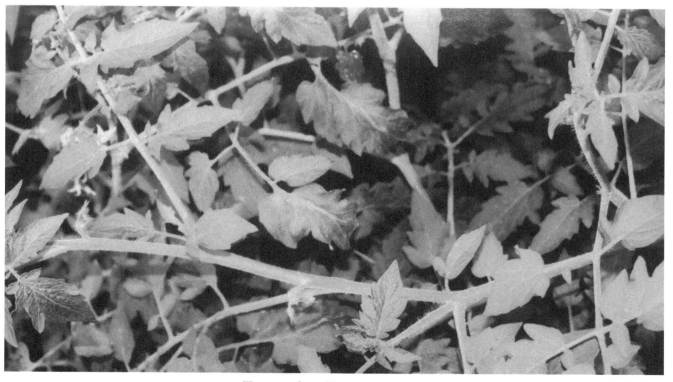

Tomato plant (*Lycopescium* spp.)

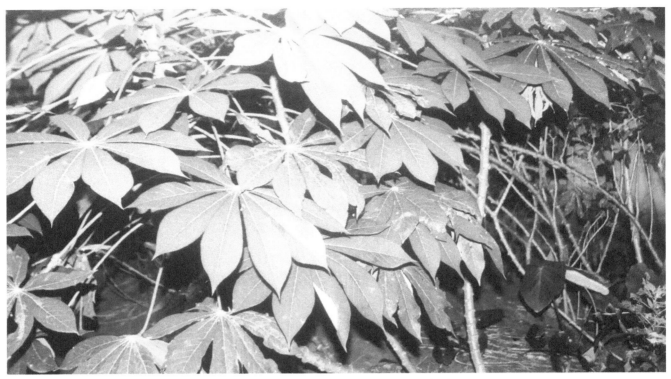

Akpu (Igbo name) (*Cassava* spp.) plant, also called *Yucca* spp

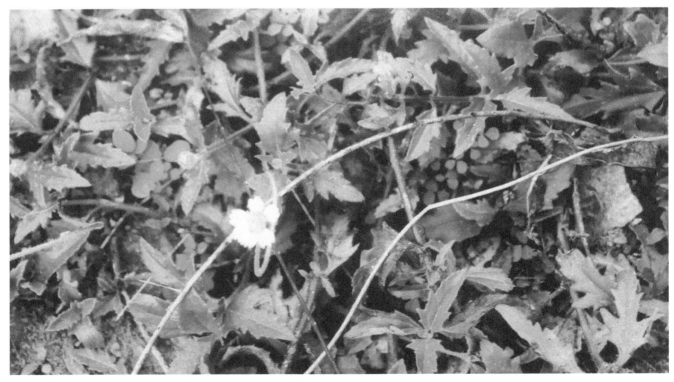

Tridax spp. plant.

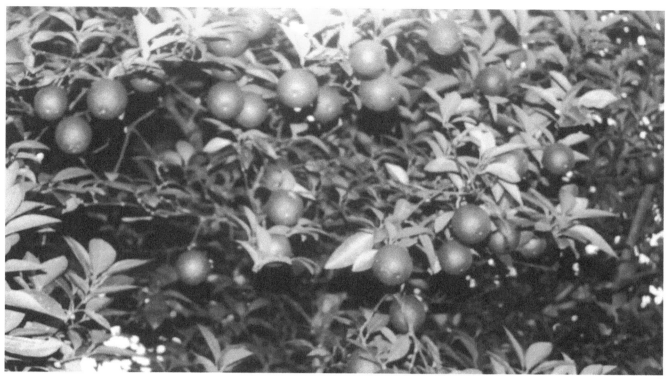

Oroma (Igbo name) or orange (*Citrus* spp.) plant

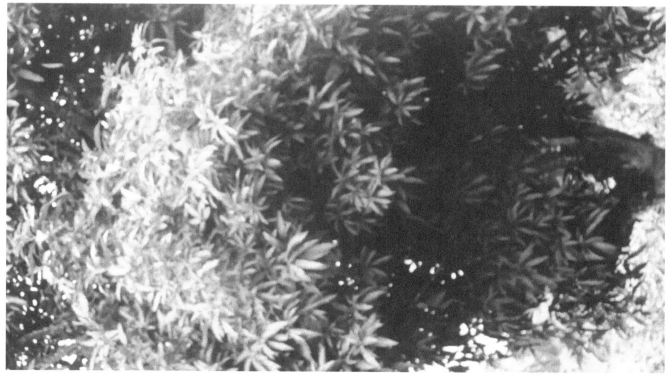

Mango tree (*Magnifera indica* spp.)

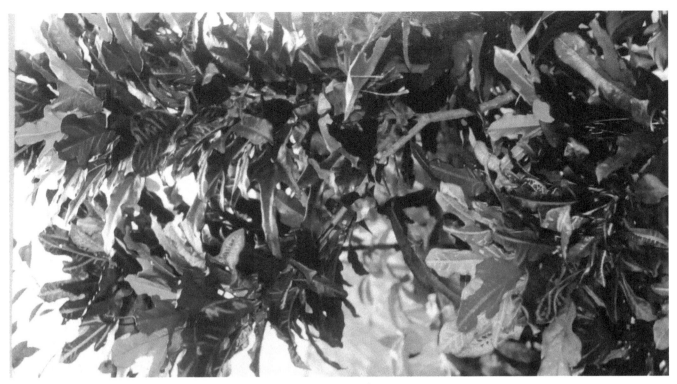

Croton spp. plant

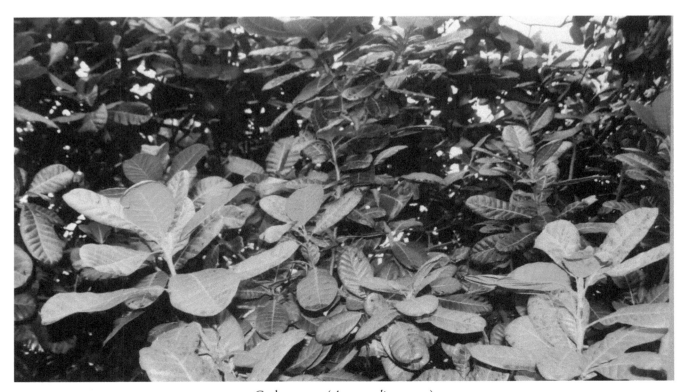

Cashew tree (*Anarcardium* spp.)

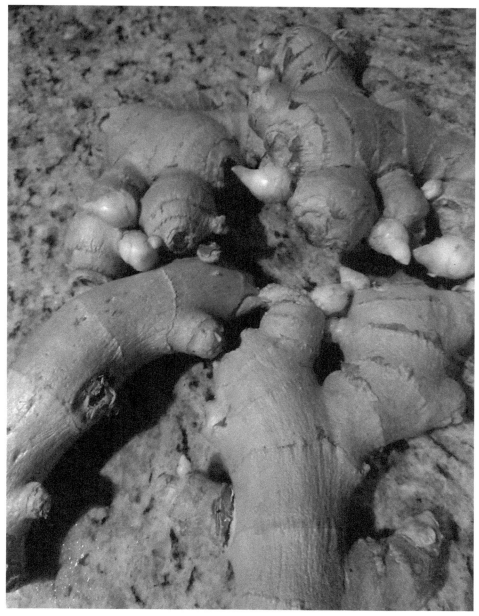

Zingiber officinale (ginger stem [rhizome])

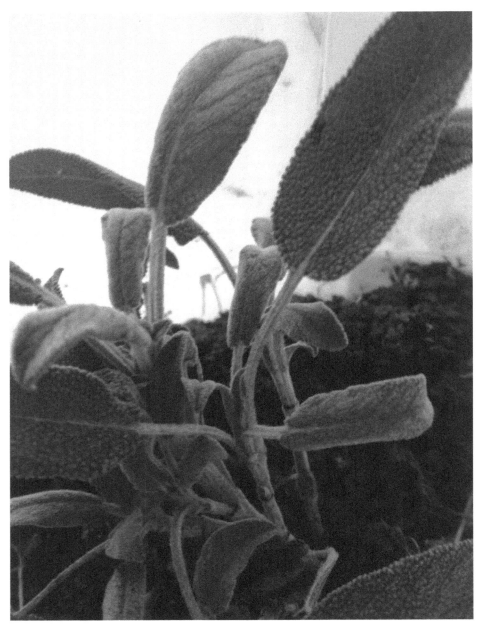

Salvia officinalis (sage)

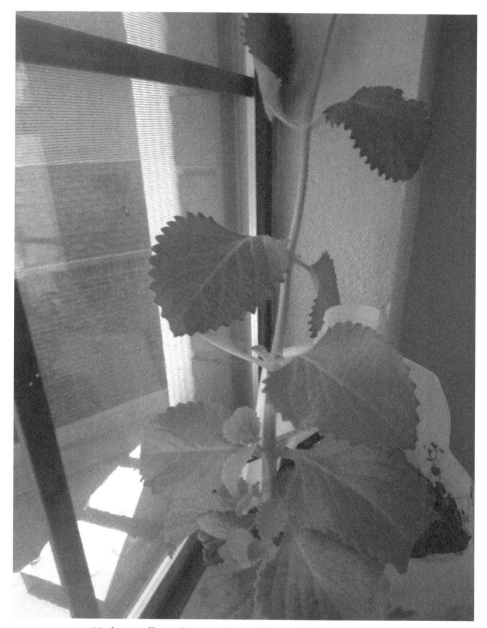

Verbena officinalis or verbena (also called vervain) herb

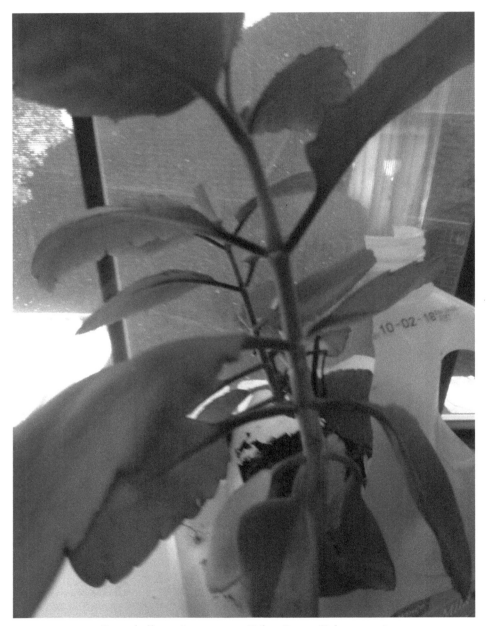

Bryophyllum pinnatum or Odaa Opuo (Igbo name)

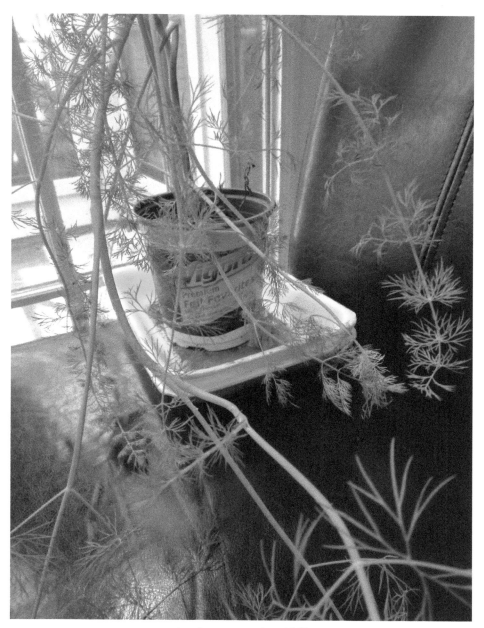

Anethum graveolens (dill)

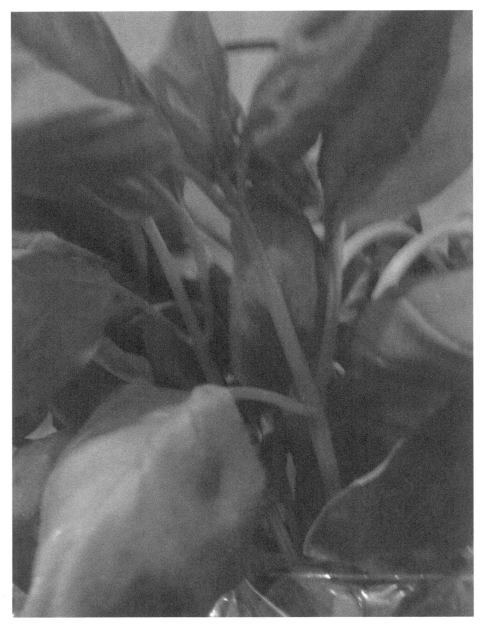

Ocimum basil (basil)

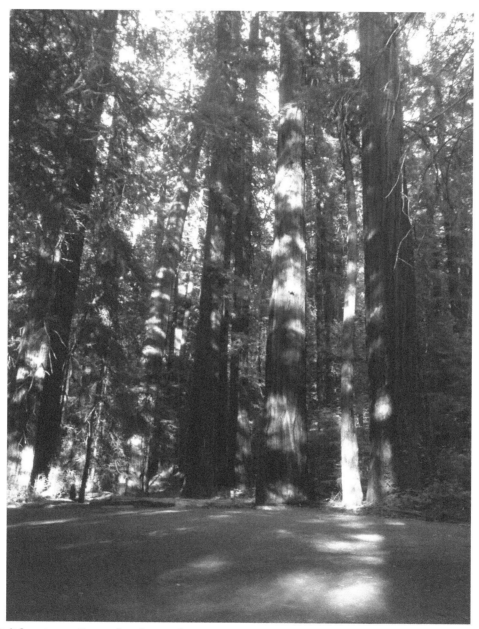

California or Coastal red wood trees, *Sequoia sempervirens* (Family *Cupressaceae*), monoecious coniferous trees that live 1,200–2,200 years.

CHAPTER 2

Which Parts of Plants Produce Medicinal Effects?

VARIOUS KINDS OF products and by-products of metabolism appear in plant cells and tissues as reserve materials, secretory products, waste products, or for the defense of plants against disease and injury. Such products may appear in the cytoplasm; in cell walls; or in the vacuoles in the cytoplasm of cells of medicinal plants. Any of such products and by-products of metabolism may demonstrate pharmacological and medicinal effects when examined. Before discussing such potential medicinal plant constituents, the basic nature and structural organization of living organisms will be summarized below.

Basic Nature and Structure of Living Things

All living organisms, whether of animal or plant origin, are made of units called cells. The essential common characteristic of living things is that they are made of a living substance called protoplasm. Body cells of an organism are therefore small but definite units of protoplasm. The protoplasm of a cell is usually divided into an inner and often centrally located smaller portion that usually contains the genetic materials of the cell called the nucleus and an outer larger portion called the cytoplasm. The nucleus usually controls the activity of the cell while the cytoplasm is the seat of most of the metabolic activities of the cell.

The protoplasm of a cell is usually delimited by a cell membrane in the case of animal cells and by a cellulose cell wall in the case of plant cells. Many subunits of protoplasm called organelles are located in the cytoplasm. Organelles act as sites of performance of specific functions by the cell and often have their own delimiting membranes. Two examples of such organelles are mitochondria, which act as the powerhouse of the cell, and the rough endoplasmic reticulum, which acts as a site of protein synthesis.

The differences between organisms appear to lie in the slight differences in their protoplasm, especially in the differences in their gene makeup, because the genes that are the essential parts of the genetic material that lies in the nucleus of a cell directs the nature of the structure and biochemical composition of substances that are used to carry out the activities of a cell, a tissue, or organ.

Constituents of Protoplasm

Gross analysis of dead protoplasm gives percentages of the various constituents of 10%–15% of its living substance because it has been found that in living protoplasm there is normally 85%–90% of water. In special conditions such as in dormant seeds and spores, the water content of their cells may fall as low as 10%.

Gross analysis of the protoplasm of a myxomycete fungus gave the following composition; water-soluble constituents: monosaccharide sugars, 14%; proteins, 2%; amino acids, 24%; inorganic salts, 4%; insoluble constituents: nucleoprotein, 32%; free nucleic acid, 3%; protein, 1%; lipoprotein, 5%; neutral fats, 7%; sterols, 3%; phosphatides, 1%; polysaccharides; pigments, etc., 4%. This shows that the protoplasm of living organisms contains both soluble and insoluble constituents, all of which constantly interact to carry out the processes that keep that organism alive.

The protoplasm is thus a colloidal structure in a state of dynamic equilibrium. The total proteins, fats, fatty acids, and inorganic salts in solution and the enzymes and intermediate metabolites of the protoplasm of a cell will always depend on the state of the multiplicity of changes constantly taking place to maintain the life of the organism. The nucleoplasm is usually acid, the cytoplasm usually a little removed from neutral, and the protoplasm almost always slightly acid.

The Effect of Medicinal Plants on Body Cells and Body Organs

Medicinal effects of orthodox drugs and medicinal plant extracts aim at normalizing the deranged, disorganized, injured, or destabilized protoplasm of tissues, organs, or organ systems of an organism. Medicines and medicinal extracts of plants essentially supply missing parts of protoplasmic activity; repair damaged tissues of an organism and/or kill or inhibit tissue-damaging effects of invading pathogenic organisms or of antigenic substances. Sometimes drugs or medicinal plant extracts simply supply the body with optimum health-promoting micronutrients or medicinal constituents.

The maintenance of the ceaseless activities that maintain the life of an organism by protoplasm is tied to the continuous supply of energy to do work, to the cell. Within the protoplasm, the energy is used to do chemical and physical work, and any excess is stored for future use as potential energy in chemical compounds like adenosine triphosphate. In the same way, the activities of medicines or plant medicinal extracts are often tied to those of the stored potential energy-bearing chemical compounds in the protoplasm of the organism that the medicine acts on.

Plant Substances That Produce Medicinal Effects

Plant substances that possess and/or demonstrate medicinal properties come from the vast ergastic substances produced by the plant body as reserve, secretory, waste, or body protective substances.

Secretory Products of Plants and Animals

Pigments of Living Organisms

Most living things produce colored substances, some of which interact with light; protect the organism from light; enable the organism to camouflage itself; is used for mimicry; or enable the organism to carry out specific physiological functions. Some secretary products of living organisms serve for the attraction of other organisms to the plant or animal in question. Examples of such pigments produced by living organisms include linear tetrapyrroles, cyclic tetrapyrroles, carotenoids, flavins, melanins, pteridines, anthocyanins, and anthoxanthins. Pigments secreted by living organisms include the purplish-red pigment of red onion leaf; the yellow pigment of carrot roots, the yellow pigment of turmeric; the red pigment of *Hibiscus sobdarifa* flowers, cherry fruit (figure 2), tomato fruits and the skin of some mango fruits; the green pigment of avocado pea flesh and many leafy vegetables; the brown pigment of nutmeg seed; and the orange or red pigment of watermelon flesh; et cetera.

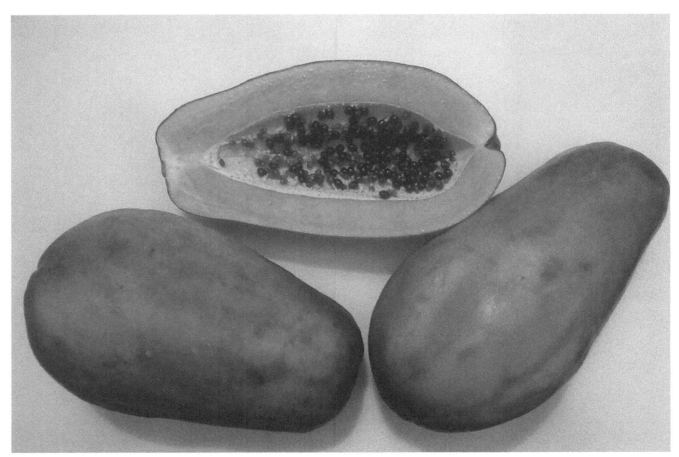

Figure 1. Some ripe pawpaw (papaya) fruits contain yellow pigment while some ripe pawpaw fruits contain a red pigment that resembles tomato fruit red pigment.

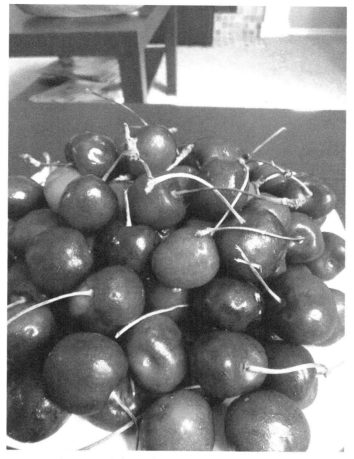

Figure 2. The red pigment of cherry fruit.

Linear tetrapyrroles are made from a skeleton formed by a chain of four pyrrole rings. Examples of linear tetrapyrroles are bilirubin ($C_{33}H_{36}O_6N_4$) and biliverdin ($C_{33}H_{34}O_6N_4$).

The cytochromes which are chromoproteins and also heme derivatives containing iron as acceptors of hydrogen from other substances are cyclic tetrapyrroles. The degree of respiratory activity in a cell roughly corresponds to the amount of cytochrome in that cell. The iron-containing red hemoglobin of vertebrates, the iron-containing red erythrocruorin of many annelids and mollusks, and the copper-containing blue hemocyanin of many mollusks and arthropods are all tetrapyrroles that serve as respiratory pigments that form oxy-derivatives by the molecular union of oxygen with the metal.

The chlorophylls a ($C_{55}H_{72}O_5N_4Mg$) and b ($C_{55}H_{72}O_6N_4Mg$), which are also cyclic tetrapyrroles, play an important role in trapping and utilization of sunlight for photosynthesis in food-producing green plants.

Carotenoids

The carotenoids include carotenes and xanthophylls. The carotenes are isomeric hydrocarbon oils with the formula $C_{40}H_{56}$. The best-known carotenes are α-carotene, β-carotene, and lycopene. Plant sources like ripe papaw fruit (figure 1), yellow carrots, and yellow chili pepper pods are good sources of carotenes. Ripe red tomatoes contain lycopene as its coloring pigment.

Hydrolysis of β-carotene yields two molecules of vitamin A, thus

$$C_{40}H_{56} + 4H_2O > C_{20}H_{30} + 4H_2$$

On the other hand, hydrolysis of α-carotene yields only one molecule of vitamin A. Since vitamin A has not been found in plants and animals make it from the carotene in the diet, carotene is sometimes called provitamin A.

Xanthophylls

Xanthophylls are hydroxyl-, carboxylic acid-, ketone-, and aldehyde- derivatives of carotenes. An example of these is the chromoprotein coloring the carapace of many crustacea red, purple, green, and blue. Chromoplasts containing carotenoids color many flowers, fruits, and seeds of plants like yellow of ripe orange and yellow of ripe cantaloupe.

The skin of some animals contains carotenoids coupled to melanin, and some such animals can lighten or darken the color of their skin and/or hair by concentration or dispersion of these colors.

Some animal and plant products like egg yolk, butter, yellow bird plumage, mangoes, etc., are yellow due to the presence of carotenoids.

Flavins

The flavins are enzymes or coenzymes involved in cell redox reactions. They are probably similar to the enzyme riboflavin. They readily accept hydrogen and thus oxidize the substrate. In the reduced state, they lose their color and regain their color when they get re-oxidized.

Pteridines

Some insect pigments are derived from the pteridine double ring. Leupterin of the wing of cabbage butterfly is an example, and xanthopterin is present in the yellow band on the wings of the wasp.

Organic Acids

Many organic acids exist free in organisms. Examples of these organic acids are dibasic non-hydroxy acids: oxalic acid, $(COOH)_2$; malonic acid, $CH_2(COOH)_2$; succinic acid, $(CH_2)_2(COOH)_2$; glutaric acid, $(CH_2)_3(COOH)_2$; adipic acid, $(CH_2)_4(COOH)_2$; fumaric acid, $(CH_2)_2(COOH)_2 CH_2)_2(COOH)_2$; cis-Aconitic acid, $CH_2CHC(COOH)_3$; hydroxy acids: glycolic acid $CH_2(OH)COOH$; lactic acid, $CH_3CH(OH)COOH$; malic acid, $CH(OH)CH_2(COOH)_2$; tartaric acid, $(CHOH)_2(COOH)_2$; citric acid, $CH_2(COH)(COOH)_3$; keto acids: pyruvic acid, $CH_3COCOOH$; oxaloacetic acid, $CH_2CO(COOH)_2$; α-ketoglutaric acid, $(CH_2)_2CO(COOH)_2$ and oxalosuccinic acid, $CH_2CHCO(COOH)_3$.

Many of the organic acids like citric, tartaric, malic, succinic, and glycolic acids are present in sour unripe fruits. These organic acids probably play a role in the regulation of the pH of such fruits while the fruits are still unripe.

The keto acids play important roles in metabolism. For example, pyruvic acid plays a key role in the respiratory energy generation of the carboxylic acid cycle or Krebs cycle. Succinic and glutaric acids, on the other hand, play key roles in the synthesis of proteins.

Fats, Oils, and Miscellaneous Compounds

Fats and oils are found in almost all plants in the form of minute globules in the protoplasm where they are formed. Fats and oils are made of carbon, hydrogen, and oxygen; but the hydrogen and oxygen are not in the same proportion as in water (unlike in carbohydrates where the carbon, hydrogen, and oxygen are in the same proportions as in water).

Fats are synthesized from fatty acids and glycerine under the influence of lipase. The fatty acids and glycerine utilized in fat synthesis are obtained from palmitic, oleic, and stearic acids generated from carbohydrate diet. In many flowering plants, special deposits of fats and oils are often found in seeds and fruits, as food the plant has stored for future use (during periods in the life cycle of the plant during which the plant is not actively producing food).

Examples of plant oils of economic importance are: olive oil; sesame oil; castor oil; linseed oil; soya bean seed oil; granola oil; coconut oil; cottonseed oil; mustard oil and groundnut or pea nut oil.

Oils are classed into two types: fixed or nonvolatile oils and essential or volatile oils.

Essential Oils

Essential or volatile oils usually occur in oil glands in plants. Essential oils are seen as transparent spots in the rind of fruits like orange, lemon, lime (figure 3) and shaddock. They also occur as transparent spots in the leaves of lemon, lemongrass, orange, eucalyptus, sacred basil, pummelo, shaddock, and in petals of flowers of many plants like rose, jasmines, etc. Volatile oils produced by plants of the family Labiatae are peppermint, spearmint, thyme, lavender, marjoram, sage, rosemary, and basil oils.

Essential oils are obtained from plant sources by distillation while fixed oils can be obtained by mere pressure. Volatile oils are soluble in alcohol but fixed oils are not. Volatile oils are sufficiently soluble in water to impart their taste and odor. Volatile oils differ from fixed oils in their chemical composition and in being volatile in steam.

Except oils derived from glycosides like bitter almond oil and mustard oil, essential oils are mixtures of hydrocarbons and oxygenated compounds derived from these hydrocarbons, but usually one compound dominates and gives the oil its characteristic scent. In some oils like oil of turpentine, the hydrocarbons predominate while in some others like oil of cloves, oxygenated compounds predominate.

The odour and taste of volatile oils are mainly determined by their oxygenated compounds that are, to some extent, soluble in water but more soluble in alcohol. Some of the compounds are derived from benzene, and some are derived from cyclohexane. A small number of oils like those of cinnamon and clove contain mainly aromatic (benzene) derivatives mixed with the terpenes. On the other hand, many oils are terpenoids in origin. Then again, a few compounds, though aromatic in structure, are terpenoid in origin.

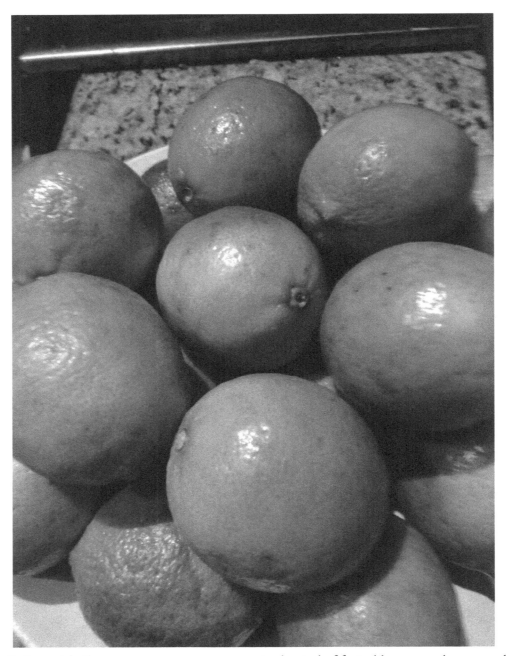

Figure 3. Essential oils are seen as transparent spots in the rind of fruits like orange, lemon, and lime.

The main constituent of a volatile oil may be terpenes or sesquiterpenes, alcohols, esters and alcohols, aldehydes, ketones, phenols, ethers, or peroxides. A volatile oil may also be nonterpenoid and derived from glycosides like mustard oil, bitter almond oil, and oil of wintergreen.

The two main groups of compounds that form the constituent of many volatile oils are the terpenes derived from cyclohexane and the camphors, which are derivatives of terpenes. Some common oils and their essential oil constituents include the following:

1. Eucalyptus oil derived from *Eucalyptus* species, which has pinene and cineole as its main constituents.
2. Cinnamon oil derived from the bark of *Cinnamomum verum*, which contains 60%–75% cinnamic aldehyde, eugenol, and terpenes. Cinnamon leaf of the same plant contains mainly eugenol (80%).
3. Oil of turpentine derived from coniferous trees contains terpenes (pinene, limonene, dipentine, and comphene).
4. Aniseed oil derived from *Pimpinella anisum* consists of 90% anethole and chavicol methyl ether, etc.
5. Attar of roses oil derived from *Rosa damascene* contains mainly geraniol and citronellol.
6. Oil of wintergreen derived from *Gaultheria* spp. contains mainly methyl salicylate.
7. Coriander oil derived from *Coriandrum sativum* contains linalool (65%–80% alcohol) and terpene.
8. Sandalwood oil from *Santalum album* contains α-Santalol (sesquiterpene alcohols), esters, and aldehydes.
9. Spearmint oil from *Mentha spicata* and *Mentha cardiaca* contains 55%–70% carvone, limonene, and esters.
10. Thyme oil from *Thymus vulgaris* contains 20–30% thymol.
11. Clove oil from *Syzygium aromaticum* contains 85%–90% eugenol, acetyl eugenol, methyl pentyl ketone, and vanillin.
12. Nutmeg oil from *Myristica fragrans* contains 60%–85% terpenes, myristicin (methoxysafrole) up to 4%, alcohols, and phenols.
13. Camphor from *Cinnamomum camphora* contains ketone, safrole, and terpenes.
14. Chenopodium oil from *Chenopodium anthelmitica* contains 60%–77% ascaridole and an unsaturated terpene peroxide.
15. Lemon oil from *Citrus limon* contains 90% limonene and about 4% citral.
16. Bitter almond oil from *Prunus communis* contains benzaldehyde and HCN from amygdalin.
17. Sage oil from *Salvia officinalis* contains 50% thujone, camphor, and cineole.
18. Lemongrass oil from *Cymbopogon* spp. contains 75%–85% citral, citronellal, and terpenes.
19. Rosemary oil from *Rosemarinus officinalis* contains 10%–18% borneol, linalool, 2%–5% bornyl acetate, terpenes, and cineole.
20. Tea tree oil from *Melaleuca alternifolia* contains cyclic monoterpenes.
21. Code oil or juniper tar oil from *Juniperus communis* contains sesquiterpenes (codeine) and phenols (guaiacol, cresol).
22. Mustard oil from *Brassica* spp. contains glucosinolates.
23. Coriander oil from *Coriandrum sativum* contains 65%–80% linalol (alcohols) and terpenes.
24. Fennel oil from *Foeniculum vulgare* contains 60% anethol and 20% fencone.
25. Dill oil from *Anethum graviolens* contains 50% carvone, limonene, etc.
26. Peppermint oil from *Mentha piperita* contains about 45% menthol and 4–9% menthyl acetate.
27. Parsley oil from *Petroselinum sativum* contains apiole (dimethoxysafrole).
28. Caraway oil from *Carum carvi* contains 60% carvone, limonene, etc.
29. Otto of rose from *Rosa* spp. contains 70%–75% alcohols geraniol, citronellol, and esters.
30. Wormwood oil from *Artemisia absinthium* contains 35% thujone, thujyl alcohol, and azulenes.

Uses of Volatile Oils

Essential oils seem to play the following roles:

1. Limiting transpiration especially in the dry season;
2. Attracting insects to the plant for pollination of its flowers; and
3. Performing medicinal roles like protecting the plant against fungal attacks and other diseases or injury.

Human uses of volatile oils include the following:

1. Use as therapeutic agents;
2. Use for flavoring foods and drinks;
3. Use in making perfumes;
4. Use as starting materials for the synthesis of other compounds.

Use of Volatile Oils as Therapeutic Agents

Volatile oils are used singly or in admixture in aromatherapy. Drops of oil are added to bathwater and mixed vigorously. Oils used transdermally in aromatherapy include oils of black pepper; benzoin, German chamomile, fennel, eucalyptus, frankincense, clove, cinnamon leaf, myrrh, orange, neroli, sandalwood, lemon, peppermint, thyme, tea tree, pine, spearmint, juniper berry, lavender, ginger, bergamot, and rosemary.

Use of Volatile Oils as Compresses

Volatile oils are also used in compresses. The volatile oils are mixed with a suitable carrier like the fixed oil of evening primrose; sweet almond; apricot kernel; palm kernel oil etc. and applied as a compress at the afflicted body part.

Use of Volatile Oils as Inhalational Drugs

Essential oils like eucalyptus oil are used as inhalations through the traditional steam inhalation method in which the face is put over a hot vapor rising from the medicinal oil with a heavy cloth placed over the head. To minimize escape of the inhalational oil into the atmosphere, a medicinal volatile oil is sometimes applied through porous materials like handkerchiefs or tissue or applied with vaporizers.

Volatile oils like peppermint oil are also used as mouth gaggles and oils like thyme oil (thymol) are present in mouthwashes.

Use of Volatile Oils as Antiseptics

Volatile oils that have high phenolic content like thyme oil and clove oil are used for antiseptic purposes.

Some volatile oils like rosemary, chamomile, peppermint, fennel, caraway, and lime (*Citrus aurantifolia*) oils show antispasmodic properties and as such are used therapeutically for this purpose.

Use of Volatile Oils as Food or Drink Preservatives

The volatile oils that demonstrate antispasmodic properties and/or demonstrate interference with respiration and electron transport in bacteria like lime oil are used in food preservation and cosmetics preparation.

Gums

Gums are generally produced by a plant's response to injury or disease of a part of the body of the plant. Plants also seem to use the gum they produce to protect the plant body from unfavorable conditions such as drought. Examples of gums are gum arabic from acacia and gum tragacanth from *Astragalus* spp. Gums and mucilages have similar constituents. On hydrolysis, gums and mucilages yield pentoses, hexoses, and uronic acids.

Gums are formed extracellularly while mucilages are formed intracellularly. Mucilages abound in okra stem and leaves or okra fruits. The cotyledons of *Irvangia* seed contain large quantities of mucilage. Large quantities of gums are formed at injured sites of stem bark of *Eucalyptus* spp. trees or stem bark of African *Persea* spp. trees. Gums are also formed in the barks of mango (*Magnifera indica*) trees.

Tragacanth Gum

Tragacanth is the air-dried gummy exudate flowing naturally or through incision of the branches and trunk of *Astragalus gummifera*. Tragacanth gum exudes immediately after injury to the plant, but gum arabic from acacia is slowly produced after injury.

Uses of Tragacanth Gum

Tragacanth gum is used in pharmacy as a suspending agent for insoluble powders and as a binding agent for medicinal tablets and pills.

Other Gums

Chitral Gum

Chitral gum is obtained from *Astragalus strobiferus*. Sterculia or karaya gum is the dried gummy exudate obtained from the Indian, Pakistani, and African tree *Sterculia urens* (family *Sterculiaceae*) which is used as a substitute or adulterant of tragacanth.

Guar Gum

Guar gum is obtained from the ground endosperm of the Indian leguminous plant, *Cyamopsis tetragonolobus*. This gum readily forms mucilage with water.

Xanthan Gum

Xantan gum is artificially produced by the fermentation action of the bacterium *Xanthomonas compestris* on glucose. Xanthan gum is used in food and pharmaceutical and cosmetic industries.

Dextran

Dextran, which is used as a plasma expander and as an absorbent in biochemical analysis, is produced like xanthan gum by the action of *klebsiella*, *acetobacter*, *Leuconostoc*, and *streptococci* on glucose.

Latex

Latex is the milky substance secreted by some plants that often contain irritating and poisonous substances. The latex of some trees produce inflammation and/or blisters when it comes in contact with skin.

Papaw plant, especially its unripe fruits; poppies like opium poppy, prickly poppy, and garden poppy; and some plants of family *Compositae* contain latex in vessels. Plants like periwinkle (*Vinca* spp.), fig and banyan (*Ficus* spp.), oleander (*Nerium* and *Thevetia* spps.), madar (*Calatropis* spp.), and spurges have their latex in latex cells.

Latex from green unripe pawpaw fruit or green pawpaw leaves is antimicrobial. The irritating and poisonous substances contained in the latex of plants seem to be for the defense of the plant against injury and infection and as such often confer such benefits when employed medicinally.

Resins and Balsams

Resins are amorphous complex plant products that soften and finally melt upon being heated. They are usually insoluble in water and petroleum spirit but soluble in alcohol, chloroform, and ether.

Resins are made of mixtures of resin acids, resin alcohols (resinols), resin phenols (resinotannols), esters, and chemically inert substances called resenes. The most important resin acid is abietic acid, $C_{19}H_{29}(COOH)$, which is made up mainly of four isoprene units.

Examples of resins are dammar from many Malayan trees, rosin from pine exudates, dragon's blood from the rattan palm, the fossil amber from *Pinites succinifer*, copal from *Hymenoea* spp. of South America, and myrrh from *Commiphora* spp.

Resins are often associated with volatile oils (oleoresins), examples of which are Canada turpentine and copaiba. Resins associated with gums are called gum-resins and resins associated with both oil and gum are oleo gum resins. Resins can be in glycosidic combination with sugars as in products obtained from plants of the family *Convolvulaceae*.

Balsams

Balsams, which are like liquid gums, are usually contained in schizogenous and schizolysigenous ducts or cavities in plants. They are often preformed products in the plant but their yield is increased by injury as seen in *Pinus* species. Examples of balsam are gum benzoin from *Strrax* spp., frankincense from *Bosweellia* spp., and Canada balsam from *Abies balsamea*. Many balsams like balsam of Tolu are not formed by the plant until it is injured suggesting that they are of pathological origin.

The balsams are usually partly soluble in hot water if they contain free acids like benzoic and cinnamic acid. Benzoin is best described as balsamic resin.

Rubber, resin, and balsam seem to protect the plant against injury, microbial attack, and physiological insults as suggested by their exudation at wounds.

Tannins

Tannins are glycosides composed of glucose combined with different phenols and hydroxyl acids. Gallotannin, the most important tannin, is made of one molecule of glucose and five molecules of digallic acid ($C_{14}H_{10}O_9$).

Commercial tannins are mixtures of tannins obtained from various trees. Tannins act on the hides of skins of animals by precipitation of proteins in the hide to form leather. Thus tannins are those substances produced by plants that can combine with the protein of animal hides to prevent their putrefaction and thus convert the hides into leather. Tannins are detected by a "tanning test." Most tannins are of molecular weight 1000 to 5000.

Many tannins are glycosides. Tannins are also seen as polyphenols illustrating particular aspects of gallic and flavan-3-ol phytochemistry. Two main types of tannins are recognizable: hydrolyzable tannins and complex tannins.

Hydrolyzable Tannins

Hydrolyzable tannins can be hydrolyzed by enzymes like tannase. Hydrolyzable tannins are formed from several molecules of phenolic acids like gallic and hexahydroxydiphenic acids, which are united to a central glucose molecule by ester linkages. The two types of hydrolyzable tannins are gallitannins and ellagitannins formed from gallic and hexahydroxydiphenic acid units. Examples of medicinal plants that contain hydrolyzable tannins are pomegranate, oak bark, and *Rosa* spp.

Condensed Tannins

Condensed tannins do not contain a sugar moiety and are not readily hydrolyzable into simpler molecules. Condensed tannins are related to the flavonoid pigments and have polymeric flavan-3-ol structures.

Condensed tannins have monomeric, dimeric, and trimeric forms. Examples of medicinal plants that contain condensed tannins are cinnamon, *Cinchona*, wild cherry, hawthorn, cranberry, grapes (figure 4), cocoa, guarana, acacia, mangrove, eucalyptus, mimosa, and willow.

Tannins may be protective of the plant and may serve medicinal, organ-protective roles. Tannins may even have protein-precipitating effects on other organisms.

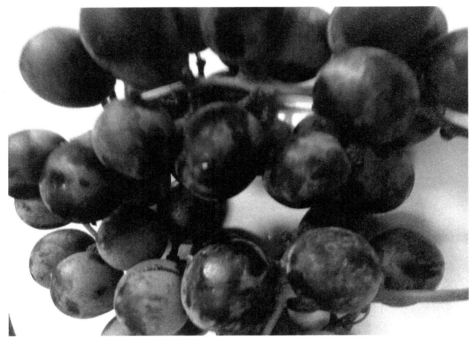

Figure 4. Black grapes. Grape trees are one of the examples of medicinal plants that contain condensed tannins.

Lignin

Lignin is a colloidal polymer derived from coniferyl alcohol. Cell walls of certain plant tissues like tracheids of xylem vessels, sclerenchyma fibers, and sclereids suddenly become impregnated with lignin on maturity, conferring greater strength and protection to these parts.

Alkaloids

Alkaloids seem to be one of the devices of defense of plants. In many cases, alkaloids are extremely poisonous, and a small quantity of some alkaloids is sufficient to kill a strong animal. For example, the alkaloid strychnine obtained from the seeds of the plant *Strychnos nux vomica* exerts a predominant effect on the spinal cord that lowers the threshold of excitability of various neurons so that any sudden stimulation of the animal to which it has been administered, with a stimulus such as noise, precipitates a tonic extensor seizure. Another alkaloid, d-tubocurarine, the active principle of the roots of *Chondodendron tomentosu*, produces flaccid paralysis of the extremities which enabled Native American wildlife hunters to catch the animal they shut with the arrow poisoned with the plant preparation containing the alkaloid.

Other examples of alkaloids are morphine in opium poppy, nicotine in tobacco, quinine in *Cinchona*, and daturine in Datura.

All alkaloids are derived from four parent heterocyclic ring structures that include pyrrole, pyridine, tropane, and quinoline. Alkaloids usually occur as salts of malic, citric, and succinic acids. Only a few plants contain alkaloids. Among these few plants are plants of these three families: *Papaveraceae*, *Ranunclaceae*, and *Solanaceae*. Alkaloids may have a nitrogen atom that may be primary as in mescaline, secondary as in ephedrine, tertiary as in atropine, or quaternary as in tubocurarine.

The pyridine alkaloids include nicotine from *Nicotiana tabacum* and piperidine from *Piper nigrum*. The main pyrrole alkaloids are stachydrine from *Stachys* spp. and pyrrolidine from carrot leaves. Tropane alkaloids include hyoscyamine from *Atropa belladonna*, atropine and hyoscine from *Datura* spp. and *Hyoscyamus* spp., and cocaine from the coca plant *Erythroxylon*.

Quinoline alkaloids include strychnine, curine, curarine from *Strychnos* spp., and quinine from *Cinchona* spp. The isoquinoline alkaloids include morphine, codeine, opium from *Papaver somniferum*, and colchicine from *Colchicum autumnale*.

The poisonous nature of alkaloids suggests their protective role for the plant against invading organisms and that their medicinal use must be in extremely minute quantities.

Glycosides

Glycosides are varied combinations of sugars and aglycones (phenol, anthraquinones, and sterols). All glycosides contain a sugar unit. However, the aglycones in the molecule of glycosides vary so much in their physical, chemical, and pharmacological properties that glycosides are classified according to the aglycone fragment with which they often occur in the plant. Thus a glycoside may be called a phenol glycoside or an anthraquinone glycoside. Glycosides are also sometimes classed according to their physical characteristics (e.g., as soap-like [as a saponin]) or according to their pharmacological actions (e.g., as a cardiac glycoside) or according to the chemical action they produce (e.g., as a cryogenic glycoside [glycoside that produces hydrocyanic acid]).

Examples of glycoside include salicin, strophanthin, senegin, and aloin. Glycosides are formed by the interaction of nucleotide glycosides like uridine diphosphate glucose (UDP-glucose) with the alcoholic or phenolic group of a second compound (through O-linkage). Such glycosides are called O-glycosides. Some other glycosides are linked through sulfur (S-linkage), carbon (C-linkage), or nitrogen (N-linkage).

Amines and Amides

Amines are very simple organic compounds visualized as derivatives of ammonia by substitution of the hydrogen atoms of ammonia. Examples are methyl amines which can be monomethylamine, CH_3NH_2; dimethylamine, $(CH_3)_2NH$; and trimethylamine $(CH_3)_3N$.

Amines occur in many plant species and the various proportions in which they occur are thought to be characteristic of species suggesting their importance in maintaining the specificity of species. Tetramethylene diamine which is also called putrescine $(NH_2).(CH_2)_4NH_2$ is produced by decaying animal protein and is derived from the amino acid ornithine. The amino acids arginine and canavanine contain the amine guanidine.

The amine betaine, $C_5H_{11}O_2N$, is found in some *Solanaceae* and *Chenopodiaceae*, and the amine trigonelline is found in potato, dahlia, and seeds of some legumes. The vitamin nicotinamide is derived from trigonelline.

Amides

Amides are derived from carboxylic acids by replacement of the -OH group with the amino group $-NH_2$. Acetic acid thus yields acetamide, glutamic acid yields glutamine, and aspartic acid yields asparagine.

Phytohormones

Plant, like animals produce hormones called phytohormones which control their metabolism.

There is strong evidence that the growth hormone is indole acetic acid. Any substance including hormones produced by plants that cause enlargement of the plant is called an auxin. Auxins seem to be abundant in the growing points of plants.

Phenols

Phenolic compounds often contain aldehydic, alcoholic, and carboxylic acid groups in addition to various phenolic acids like salicylic acid, caffeic acid, and ferulic acid. Phenolic groups commonly form glycosides with various combinations of sugars.

Simple phenolic compounds include catechol, salicylic acid, thymol, eugenol, and hydroquinone. Catechol or o-dihydroxybenzene occurs in a free state in kola seeds and the leaves of *Gaultheria* spp.

Examples of phenolic glycosides include gaultherin from *Gaultheria*; betula and salicin from *Salix* and *Populus* spps.; benzoyl-salicin from *Populus tremula*, and syringin from plants of family *Oleaceae*.

Saponins

Saponins are glycosides that have the property of producing a frothing aqueous solution. As glycosides saponins are hydrolyzed by acids to produce an aglycone (sapogenin), various sugars, and related uronic acids. Saponins are classed into steroidal (which are usually tetracyclic triterpenoids) and pentacyclic types.

Examples of saponins are dioscin from *Dioscorea* spp., digitonin, and tomatidin.

Some other constituents of plants that produce medicinal effects other than those described in this chapter will be acquainted with in subsequent chapters.

CHAPTER 3

Effects of Medicinal Plants

MUCH A LOT of scientific research have been going on for decades to establish the medicinal effects of medicinal plants on humans, animals, and plants. These effects of medicinal plants are also referred to as the pharmacological and physiological effects of the medicinal plants in the living organism to which the medicinal plant extract or its isolate or its fraction is applied. In some cases, scientific studies on medicinal plants are done to identify the phytochemical constituents of the medicinal plant extract or juice that produces these effects in living organisms to which they are applied or administered.

Chapters 3 to 7 will be devoted to presenting pharmacological and physiological effects of medicinal plants of randomly selected plant families as observed from scientific research studies on their extracts and juices.

Effects of Medicinal Plants of Family *Acanthaceae* and Family *Agavaceae* as Evidenced by Scientific Studies on Their Extracts and Juices

Family *Acanthaceae*

Plants of family *Acanthaceae* are flowering plants which include shrubs, herbs, twines, vines, and epiphytes. Most plants of family *Acanthaceae* are in tropical regions while few are in temperate regions of the world. Examples of species of *Acanthus* plants include: *Acanthus ilicifolius, Acanthus montanus, Acanthus mollis, Acanthus volubilis, and Acanthus spinosus.* The parts of plants of family *Acanthaceae* most frequently used in traditional medicine are the leaves.

> Phytochemical constituents of plants of family *Acanthaceae* include glycosides, flavonoids, benzonoids, phenolic compounds, naphthoquinone, and triterpenoids.[1]
> Various parts of the plant *Acanthus ilicifolius* have been employed in traditional medicine to treat diabetes; asthma; hepatitis; leprosy; snakebites; rheumatoid arthrities[2].
> *Acanthus ebracteatus* used in Thai and Indonesian herbal tea is known to have anti-oxidant properties[3].
> *Acanthus ilicifolius* is used in Indian and Chinese traditional medicine[4].

In India, the leaves of *Adhaoda vasica* are used as a uterine tonic and for the treatment of cough and allergies.

Some Research Studies Done on Plants of the Family Acanthaceae

The antitussive effects of *Adhaoda vasica* leave extract were demonstrated pharmacologically by Dudley in the *Journal of Ethnopharmacology* 67 (1999), page 361, and its hepatoprotective property was reported by Bhattacharyya in *Fitoterapia* 76 (2005), page 223.

A medicinal plant of Acanthaceae family, *Monechma ciliatum* is used in folk medicine of the Plateau State of Nigeria to induce labor and menses.

The methanol extract of *Monechma ciliatum* induced rhythmic contractions of rat isolated uterus and contracted other smooth muscles (rat ileum and fundus, guinea pig ileum, and rabbit duodenum) in a concentration-dependent manner, and the contractions were antagonized by atropine and potentiated by physostigmine. It also increased the twitch responses of the rat's isolated phrenic-nerve-diaphragm preparation[5] to both nerve and muscle stimulation.

In another study, methanol extract of *Monechma ciliatum* dose-dependently lowered rat blood pressure, an effect which was more prolonged than that produced by acetylcholine and was blocked by atropine.[6]

The methanol extract of *Monechma ciliatum*, when tested for oxytocic activity, contracted the nonpregnant rat uterus but not the pregnant rat uterus and demonstrated oestrogenic effects judged by uterus weight ratio, premature vaginal opening, and degree of vaginal cornification.[7]

The uterogenic activity of hot methanol extract of *Monechma ciliatum* was partially blocked by atropine, inhibited by indomethacin, and blocked by D-600, which suggested that the methanol extract of *Monechma ciliatum* acted on uterine smooth muscle through more than one mechanism.[8]

Bioassay-directed isolation of oxytocic principles from the methanol extract of *Monechma ciliatum* on rat isolated uterus suggested that the oxytocic principle that contracted nonpregnant rat uterus is a small peptide made up of tyrosine, leucine, and probably serine (which makes it comparable to oxytocin which is also a peptide with tyrosine and leucine in its structure).[10]

Four different solvent extracts of *Monechma ciliatum* showed good antibacterial activity. The petroleum ether extract showed the highest antibacterial activity against the organisms tested.[11]

Rats and mice were given 10 mg and 100 mg of aqueous extract of *Monechma ciliatum* for two weeks to investigate the toxicity potential of the extract on the food and water intake, urine, feces, blood parameters, and on liver function enzymes of the mice. The LD_{50} calculated in mice to which the extract was given by the intraperitoneal route was 3.16/kg.[12]

The study found that the extract did not affect any of the functions and parameters investigated adversely.[12]

The methanol extract of *Acanthus montanus* (6.25-100 mg/mL) concentration dependently relaxed the rabbit jejunum and inhibited its spontaneous contraction. This relaxation effect of *Achantus montanus* extract was not blocked by propranolol (3×10^{-7}M); was partially antagonized by phentolamine 10^{-6}-3×10^{-6}M, procaine (10^{-3}M), and methylene blue (10^{-5}M); and was reversed by CaC_{12} (0.1-1 mM)[9].

Procaine (10^{-3}M) and methylene blue (10^{-5}M) completely blocked the direct relaxant effects of *Acanthus montanus* extract and that of isoprenaline (10^{-8}-3×10^{-4}) on guinea pig *Taenia coli*[9].

The *Acanthus montanus* extract (0.1-1 mg/mL) shifted the concentration-response curves of CaC_{12} on guinea pig taenia coli to the right in a concentration-dependent manner[9].

The concentration-dependent relaxation of the KCl-precontracted taenia coli of the guinea pig produced by *Acanthus montanus* extract was only partially blocked by the propranolol (3×10^{-5} M), which completely blocked the relaxant effect of isoprenaline (10^{-8}-3×10^{-4}) on guinea pig *Taenia coli*[9].

These results suggest that the relaxant effects produced by *Acanthus montanus* extract on rabbit jejunum and guinea pig taenia coli were not produced through adrenergic mechanisms or on adrenergic receptors. The results also suggest that the relaxant effects produced by *Acanthus montanus* extract on rabbit jejunum and guinea pig taenia coli were produced through interaction with a combination of both α and β "adrenergic receptors" as this relaxation response of *Acanthus montanus* extract was partially blocked by phentolamine and partially blocked by propranolol. Studies of this author on chick rectum with eighteen pharmacologic agents[11, 12] revealed that serotonin receptor is the receptor that contains both α and β receptors as its constituents. So it is likely that *Acanthus montanus* extract produced is relaxation responses in the serotonin receptors of rabbit jejunum and guinea pig *Taenia coli*[9].

Another study investigated the analgesic effects of the methanol extract of *Acanthus montanus* leaf in rats using the cold-water tail-flick assay and in mice using the tail immersion, tail clip, acetic-acid-induced writhing, and formalin pain tests.[13] The results of the study showed that there were significant ($P < 0.05$) dose-dependent increases in pain threshold in treated mice and rats at sixty-minute post-treatment with 200mg/kg and 400mg/kg of the extract in the tail-flick, tail-immersion, and tail-clip methods.

The *Acanthus montanus* extract (100-400 mg/kg), also exhibited a dose-dependent inhibition of writhing and a significant ($P < 0.001$) inhibition of both phases of the formalin pain test but with a more intense effect on the second than on the first phase of the formalin test. These results suggested that *Acanthus montanus* leaf extract has analgesic properties and that these analgesic effects of *Acanthus montanus* leaf extract were both centrally and peripherally mediated.[13]

Family Agavaceae

The Agavaceae are a family of 20 genera and 670 species. Among the genera of family Agavaceae are *Yucca, Agave, Cordyline, Dracaena, Sansevieria, Phormium, Nolina,* and *Furcraea*, which contain 20, 300, 15, 150, 60, 2, 30, and 20 species respectively.

Steroidal saponins occur in species of *Yucca, Agave, Dracaena,* and *Furcraea*. Steroidal saponins have been reported as constituents of the resin of plants of family Agavaceae. *Sansevieria, Furcraea,* and *Agave* species produce gigantic hemp fibers. The fermented sap of *Agave sisalana* forms the Mexican drink pulque.

A dark-red secretion from the leaves and trunk of *Dracaena draco* and *Dracaena cinnabari* is called dragon's blood. Commercial Socotra dragon's blood, which has been shown to contain flavonoids, is produced from *Dracaena cinnabari*.

Some Research Studies Done on Plants of Family Agavaceae

Steroidal saponins in the leaves of three agave plants—*Agave Americana*, *Agave augustifolia*, and *Agave sisalana*—were analyzed by enzymatic hydrolysis. The enzymatic hydrolysis yielded free hecogenin and tigogenin quantified by gas chromatography.

Exogenous cellulose of pectinase not only replaced the endogenous enzymes in the release of tigogenin in *A. augustifolia* and *A. Sisalana*, but cellulase appeared more effective in this action.[17]

Leaves of flowering plants contained more sapogenin than those of nonflowering plants.[18] Higher yields of hecogenin were obtained from *Agave* species in the dry than in the wet seasons in eastern and western zones of Nigeria.[19]

Saponins from extracts of two West African "soap trees"—*Dracaena* spp., *Dracaena mannii*, and *Dracaena arborea*—were evaluated for biological activity with the following test systems: radio-respirometry, cytosensor bioautography, molluscicidal tests, agar dilution methods, and bioassay-directed fractionation of the methanol extract of seed pulp using a combination of chromatographic techniques (gel filtration, droplet countercurrent chromatography, and low-pressure liquid chromatography). The results of these studies were the isolation and characterization of spiroconazole A, a pennogenin triglycoside, 3-beta-O-[α-L-rhamnopyranosyl(1-2)], and α-L-rhamnopyranosyl(1->3)-beta-D-glucopyranosyl]-17-α-hydroxyl-spirost-5-ene].[20]

Spiroconazole A showed pronounced antileishmanial, antimalarial, molluscicidal properties. Spiroconazole A also demonstrated bacteriostatic activities against four species of bacteria and fungistatic or fungicidal activity against seventeen species of fungi.[21]

The antimalarial activity of the petroleum spirit, chloroform, and ethyl acetate fractions of the root and leaf water extract of *Dracaena fragrans* were evaluated on resistant HF28 chloroquine-resistant strain of *Plasmodium falciparum* in vitro using chloroquine plus verapamil as standard drugs.

The MIC value of chloroquine was 0.056 mg/mL while the MIC of chloroquine plus verapamil was 0.185 mg/mL. The MIC of the petroleum spirit, chloroform and ethyl acetate fractions of the root extract of *Dracaena fragrans* was 8.3 mg/mL. The highest dose of the extract tested, 25 mg/mL of the root extract of *D. fragrans*, showed 8.2% inhibition of the HF28 chloroquine-resistant strain of *Plasmodium falciparum* while chloroquine-verapamil combination could not inhibit this strain of *Plasmodium falciparum*.

References

1. A. J. Awan, Aslam M. S., "Family *Acanthaceae*, and Genus Aphelandra Ethnopharmacological and Phytochemical Review," *International Journal of Pharmacy and Pharmaceutical Sciences* 6, 10 (2014): 44–55.
2. W. M. Bandaranayake, "Traditional and medicinal uses of mangroves; Mangroves and Salt Marshes," 2, 3 (1998): 133–148, doi: 10, 1023/a 1009988607044 S2CID 129317332.
3. E. W. C. Chan et al., "Anti-oxidant and Sensory Properties of Thai Herbal Teas with Emphasis on *Thunbergia laurifolia* Lindl," *Chiang Mai J. Sci.* 39, 4 (2012): 599–609.
4. R. Wostmann and G. Liebez, "Chemical composition of the mangrove holly *Acanthus ilicifolius* (*Acanthaceae*)" (2008).

5. M. O. Uguru and F. K. Okwuasaba, *Proceedings of the Nigerian Society of Pharmacognocy* (1990): 86–98.

6. M. O. Uguru, F. K. Okwuasaba, and M. Ekwenchi, "The Cardiovascular and other Pharmacological Properties of the Methanol extract of *Monechma ciliatum*," *West African Journal of Pharmacology and Drug Research* 9, 10 (1991): 120.

7. M. O. Uguru et al., "Oxytocic and Oestrogenic effects of *Monechma ciliatum* Methanol Extract in in vivo and in vitro in Rodents," *Phytotherapy Research* 9 (1995): 26–291.

8. M. O. Uguru et al., "Uterotonic properties of methanol extract of *Monechma ciliatum*," *Journal of Ethnopharmacology* 62 (1998): 203–208.

9. O. O Adeyemi, S. O. Okpo, and C. C. Young-Nwafor, "The relaxant activity of the Methanol Extract of *Acanthus montanus* on Intestinal Smooth Muscles," *Journal of Ethnopharmacology* 68, 1–3 (1999): 169–173.

10. M. O. Uguru, M. M. Ekwenchi, and F. Evans, "Bioassay-directed Isolation of Oxytocic Principles from the methanol extract of *Monechma ciliatum*," *Phytotherapy Research* 13 (1999): 696–699.

11. M. O. Uguru, E. Ekundayo, and P. O. Olorunnfemi, "Investigation of the Leaves of *Monechma ciliatum* for Animicrobial Activity," *West African Journal of Biological Sciences* 11 (2000): 34–38.

12. M.O. Uguru, "Effects of *Monechma ciliatum* Extract in Mice and Rats," *African Journal of Natural Sciences* (2002): 55.

13. O. O. Adeyemi, S. O. Okpo, and O. Okpaka, "The Analgesic Effect of the Methanol Extract of *Acanthus montanus*," *Journal of Ethnopharmacology* 90 (2004): 45–48.

14. Uchechukwu Anastasia Utoh-Nedosa, "Evidence that Adrenergic; Muscarinic; Histaminic; Anti-malarial drugs; Opioid; NSAID, Nicotinic; Vasodilator drugs; Rauwolfian alkaloid and Adenosine Receptors are Parts or Whole of the Serotonin Receptor: chick rectum studies," Presented in Track 3 (Clinical Pharmacy and its Key Role in Treatment, International Summit on Clinical Pharmacy and Dispensing) (November 18–20, 2013), Hilton San Antonio Airport Hotel, Texas, USA.

15. Uchechukwu Anastasia Utoh-Nedosa, "Nicotinic receptors are 5-hydroxytryptamine Receptors: Evidence from Relaxation Effects of d-Tubocurarine and Hexamethonium on Chick rectum Smooth Muscles," Presented in Track 9–10 (Clinical Pharmacy and Drug Reactions/Clinical Drug Development and Therapeutics, International Summit on Clinical Pharmacy and Dispensing) (Nov. 18-20, 2013), Hilton San Antonio Airport Hotel, Texas, USA.

16. J. M. Agbedahusi, A. A. Elujoba, and S. K. Adesina, "Estimation of Hecogenin and Tigogenin from Nigerian *Agave* plants," *Nigerian Journal of Pharmaceutical Sciences* 3, 1 (1987): 23–28.

17. Jackson and J. D. Tally, "Biological Activity of Sapogenins from two *Dracaena* species, Advanced Experiment and Medical Sapogenins in Nigerian *Agave* and *Furcraea* species," *Fitoterapia* 68, 1 (1996).

18. C. O. Okunji, M. M. Iwu, and J. E. Biology, 404: 415–28.

19. A. A. Gbolade et al., "Factors affecting the levels of Steroidal" (1992).

20. Ibid.

21. Ibid.

CHAPTER 4

Effects of Medicinal Plants of Family *Anacardiaceae* and Family *Annonaceae*

THIS CHAPTER HIGHLIGHTS pharmacological and physiological effects of medicinal plants of family *Anacardiaceae* and family *Annonaceae* as evidenced by scientific research studies on their extracts and juices.

The Anacardiaceae are the cashew family of plants and include plants like cashew, mango, smoke tree, poison ivy, sumac, pistachio, marula, yellow mombin, and cuachalalate.[1] The double-shell covering cashew nut contains the substance urushiol, which is irritant to the skin, hazardous when its fumes are breathed in, and stains clothing. This substance is detoxified by heat. Urushiol is also present in poison ivy.

Family *Anacardiaceae* is made up of sixty genera containing about six hundred species. Poison ivy belongs to this family of plants. Some genera of *Anacardiaceae* family include *Anacardium*, *Pistacia*, *Magnifera*, *Rhus*, *Toxicodendron*, *Lannea*, *Cotinus*, and *Schinus*. Products typical of plants of this family include dyeing and tanning materials, resins, wax, and terpenoid acids.

Some Researches Done on Plants of Family *Anacardiaceae*

Extracts of the bark of *Anacardium*, *Magnifera*, and *Sclerocarya* species are used in Nigerian traditional combination phytotherapy against ailments like malaria, diabetes and skin diseases.

Phytochemical studies on the extract of the bark of *Sclerocarya birrea* (family *Anacardiaceae*) resulted in the isolation of sucrose, gallic acid, hydrolyzable tannins (20.88%), and a cholesterol ester (0.034% cholesterol).[2]

The physicochemical properties of *Magnifera indica* seed fat used as suppository base were studied. It was found that the extracted fat of *Magnifera indica* seed was cream-colored, possessed a pleasant odor, and had a pH of 5.0. It melted within 32°C–35°C and remained solid at room temperature.

The refractive index of the *Magnifera indica* seed fat was 1.4628, and its viscosity was 44.84 poise in the liquid form. The acid, iodine, saponification, and unsaponifiable mater values of the *Magnifera Magnifera* seed fat were 5.04g, 43.35g, 188g, and 1.11g respectively. In comparison with coco butter, formulation with *Magnifera indica* seed fat produced faster and more optimal release of salicylic acid.[3]

In a screening of eight Nigerian medicinal plant extracts used in Nigerian traditional medicine for antibacterial properties in vivo and in vitro using the hole-plate diffusion method, most of the extracts were active against gram-positive bacteria while only the extract of two plants (*Angeiossus schimperi* and *Anacardium occidentale* [cashew]) showed good antibacterial activity against *Escherichia coli* and *Pseudomonas aeruginosa*, which are gram-negative bacteria.[4]

The hypoglycaemic effects of the aqueous extract of the stem bark of *Sclerocarya birrea* were evaluated in normal (normoglycaemic) and streptozotocin (STZ) treated diabetic Wistar rats. The hypoglycaemic effect of graded doses of 100-800 mg/kg *Sclerocarya birrea* extract administered orally to groups of both fasted normal and fasted diabetic rats were evaluated.

A single dose of 800mg/kg of the *Sclerocarya birrea* extract was administered orally to a separate group of normoglycaemic and diabetic rats, and the hypoglycaemic effects of this 800mg/kg extract were compared with that of chlorpropamide (250mg/kg).

In a dose-dependent manner, acutely administered 100-800 mg/kg doses of the *Sclerocarya birrea* stem bark extract and chlorpropamide (250 mg/kg) significantly ($P < 0.05$-0.001) reduced blood glucose concentrations of both the fasted normal and fasted diabetic rats. On the other hand, the single-dose 800mg/kg extract at a higher level of significance ($P < 0.01$-0.001), reduced the glucose level of both the fasted normal and fasted diabetic rats.

These results show that the water extract of stem bark of *Sclerocarya birrea* possesses strong hypoglycaemic properties and lends credence to the folklore use of the extract in the management of adult-onset diabetes mellitus.[5]

A study evaluated the anti-inflammatory properties of *Sclerocarya birrea* {(A. Rich) Hochst} (family *Anacardiaceae*) stem-bark aqueous and methanol extracts (500mg/kg body weight) on rat paw edema induced by subplanter injections of fresh albumen (0.5 mL/kg) using acetylsalicylic acid (100mg/kg) as the standard anti-inflammatory agent.

Both the aqueous and methanol extracts of the stem bark of *Sclerocarya birrea* (500 mg/kg p.o.) progressively and time-dependently reduced rat paw edema, which demonstrated the anti-inflammatory properties of *Sclerocarya birrea* extract. The methanol extract showed a higher anti-inflammatory effect and acetylsalicylic acid had a more potent anti-inflammatory effect than the aqueous and methanol extracts.[6]

Effects of Plants of Family *Annonaceae*

Family *Annonaceae* contains about 120 genera and 2,100 species. Some of the genera of family *Annonaceae* are *Annona*, *Monodora*, *Uvaria*, and *Xylopia*. Plants of this family are shrubs or trees; and the fleshy mesocarp, whole fruit, or seed is often of primary food or medicinal interest. Examples of plants of this family include soursop, sweetsop, nutmeg, *Dennettia tripetala*, Ethiopian pepper (*Xylopia* spp.), calabash nutmeg, *Monodora myristica*, custard apple, and *Annona atemoya*.

Chemical constituents of members of family *Annonaceae* include alkaloids, especially of the quinoline type; flavonoids; diterpenes; triterpenes; and oleoresins.

A review of the volatile compounds found in plants of family *Annonaceae* shows that they contain more than two hundred different volatile compounds. Most of these volatile compounds are mono- and sesquiterpenoids. Examples of these compounds are α/β-pinene, p-cymene, myrcene, limonene, linalool, and 8-cineole. Some plants that contain rare volatile compounds like prenyl indoles (sesquiterpenoid) have sometimes been isolated.[7]

Research Studies on Plants of Family *Annonaceae*

Phytochemical studies on the extract of the bark of *Annona senegalensis* showed that it contained kauran-16-ol, kauran-16-en-19-oic acid, kauran-19-al-17-oic, and 19-norkauran-4-ol-17-oic, which are diterpenes.[8]

The volatile oil was obtained from *Monodora myristica* seeds by steam distillation and consisted mainly of monoterpenes and a low percentage of sesquiterpene hydrocarbons as determined by GC-MS and ^{13}CNMR. The oil did not show significant antibacterial activity against test organisms.[9]

Analysis of the essential oils of *Monodora tenuifolia* fruits by capillary gas chromatography and gas chromatography-mass spectrometry indicated the presence of thirty-six components, and thirty-three of these compounds identified constituted 84.9% of the total oil. The compounds were arranged in order of elution from an OV-351 capillary column and constituted mainly of sesquiterpene hydrocarbons (80.9%). The oil also contained a mixture of monoterpenoids (1.78%) and sesquiterpenoids (0.8%).

The predominant constituents of the sesquiterpene hydrocarbons of *Monodora tenuifolia* essential oil were ơ-elemene and germacrene-D (24.8% and 31.25% respectively). Other major sesquiterpene hydrocarbon contents of the oil were α-santalene (2.4%), β-elemene (1.8%), β-caryophyllene (2.0%), ơ-cadinene (5.9%), and Y-cadinene.[10]

The high content of sesquiterpene hydrocarbons in *tenuifolia* essential oil is suggestive of high anti-infective agents' activity.

The stem bark extract of *Enantia chlorantha Oliv* (family *Annonaceae*) produced two major known protoberberine alkaloids, palmatine chloride, and jatrorhizine chloride, in yields permitting an unambiguous assignment of their ^{13}CNMR chemical shifts from 2-D homo- and heteronuclear studies. The antimalarial potentials of these compounds against multidrug-resistant *Plasmodium falciparum* were evaluated in vitro. The results showed that stem bark extract of *Enantia chlorantha* had antimalarial activity and that the antimalarial activities were remarkably dependent on the structures of the constituent compounds.[11]

An investigation of the composition of the hydro-distilled fragrant yellowish essential oil of *Dennettia tripetalla* seed using gas chromatographic (GC) and gas chromatography-mass spectrometric (GC-MS) analyses showed that the oil contained a total of eleven constituents.[12]

Water and methanol extracts of *Xylopia aethiopicum* (family *Annonaceae*) significantly (P < 0.05) inhibited intestinal propulsive movements by 37% and prolonged mouth-colon transit time in test rats in comparison to control rats that received water only.[13] This suggests that aqueous and methanol extracts of *Xylopia aethiopicum* have antispasmodic properties.

Intraperitoneally administered aqueous extract of *Enantia chlorantha* (family Anonnaceae) (1.0-5.0 g/kg) elevated pain threshold, but the action of the extract was twenty times less potent than that of morphine.

Aqueous *Enantia chlorantha* extract (15.0 g/kg) given orally to rabbits relieved the pyrogenic induced fever in them produced by *Klebsiella* with which they had been infected, which was not observed in control rabbits.[14] These results suggest analgesic and antipyretic properties of aqueous *Enantia chloratha* extract.

The major component of the volatile oil and hexane extracts of *Dennettia tripetala*, 2-phenyl-1-nitro-ethane, was synthesized from benzaldehyde in a two-step reaction through 2-phenyl-1-nitro-ethane with an improved yield.

Two other components of *Dennettia tripetala* extract, p-nitro-2-phenyl-1-nitro-ethane and p-methoxy-2-phenyl-1-nitro-ethane, were also synthesized from their corresponding aldehydes.

Screening of these four synthesized compounds of *Dennettia tripetala* extract for antifungal activity on ten test fungi showed that all four compounds demonstrated high antifungal properties at a concentration of 200 mg/mL.

The unsubstituted nitro vinyl compound and the p-nitro vinyl derivative inhibited the growth of all ten test fungi, but the antifungal activities of the p-nitro vinyl derivative were higher than those of the unsubstituted nitro vinyl compound in most cases. The only saturated analogue, 2-phenyl-nitro-ethane, had the least MIC of 12.5 mg/mL for three of the five fungi it was only able to inhibit. The p-methoxy-nitro-vinyl derivative inhibited eight test fungi.[15]

These results demonstrated the antifungal properties of the volatile oil of *Dennettia tripetalla* seed and its chemical components that are responsible for these antifungal effects.

Aqueous extract of *Xylopia aethiopica* seeds from oral consumption of 300mg total dose by visually active volunteers lowered the intraocular pressure by 17.48%, reduced the near point of convergence by 31.1%, and increased the amplitude of accommodation by 8.98%, which are positively correlated (r = 0.95).[16] These results demonstrated antispasmodic effects of *Xylopia aethiopica* extract beneficial in the management of increased intraocular pressure.

Essential oils of *Xylopia aetiopica* showed activity against four microorganisms.[17] Other studies demonstrated antimicrobial activity of xylopic acid and other constituents of *Xylopia aethiopica*.[18] Some other studies also found that extracts of *Xylopia aethiopica* demonstrated activity against gram-positive and gram-negative bacteria[19], [20] and also against Candida albicans.[21], [22] Another study demonstrated antibacterial and antifungal activity of essential oils of *Xylopia aethopica* and *Monodora myristica*.[23]

At 5 mg/mL concentration essential oils of *Xylopia aethiopica* showed cytotoxicity to Hep-2 cell line, thereby demonstrating its cytotoxicity to carcinoma cells.[24]

Some studies have demonstrated other beneficial physiological systemic effects of *Xylopia aethiopica*. For example, a study demonstrated cardiovascular and diuretic activity and natriuretic effects of kaurene derivatives of *Xylopia aethopica* comparable to those of chlorothiazide.[11]

A study in albino rats showed that ethanol extract of dry *Xylopia* fruit has dose-dependent antipyretic activity comparable to that of paracetamol and dose-dependent anti-inflammatory activity comparable to those of indomethacin. The study also showed that the antipyretic and anti-inflammatory effects of 400 mg/kg *Xylopia* extract are higher than those of 150 mg/kg paracetamol, 100 mg/kg aspirin, and 200 mg/kg indomethacin, which justifies the use of *Xylopia* fruit extract as a frontline folk postpartum tonic for the relief of fever, headache, backache, and inflammation in postpartum conditions of women following childbirth.[23]

An evaluation of the effect of the ethanol extract of *Xylopia aethiopica* on hematological and biochemical indices in male rats showed that oral *Xylopia* extract produced significant ($P < 0.001$) augmentation of Hb (hemoglobin), total WBC (white blood cells), and neutrophils in a dose-dependent manner. The extract also dose-dependently caused a significant increase in serum total protein, albumin, globulin, high-density lipoproteins (HDL), cholesterol levels, and indirect and total bilirubin. It also caused a decreased serum ALT (alkaline transaminase enzyme). The results validated the traditional use of *Xylopia aethiopica* as an immune booster and postpartum tonic.[25]

Effects of ethanol extract of *Xylopia aethiopica* were evaluated on the male reproductive organs of Wistar rats. Three groups of Wistar rats received no extract, 0.5 mL, or 1.0 mL *Xylopia* extract once daily for twenty-eight days.

The results of the study showed a significant ($P < 0.05$) and dose-dependent decrease in the semen parameters (count and motility) and a nonsignificant decrease in the percentage of sperms with normal morphology. The photomicrographs of the small percentage of sperms with abnormal morphology showed dose-dependent degenerative changes. These results suggest that chronic administration of high doses of ethanol extract of *Xylopia aethiopica* may have an antifertility effect on the male reproductive organs of animals.[26]

Extract of *Xylopia aethiopica* prepared with 70% ethanol showed antiproliferative activity against a panel of cancer cell lines. The IC_{50} was estimated at 12 µg/mL against HCT116 colon cancer cells and 7.5 µg/mL and > 25 µg against U937 and KGIa leukemia cells.

The main cytotoxic and DNA-damaging compound in ethanol extract of Xylopia aethiopica is ent-15-oxokur-16-en-19-oic acid.[27]

References

1. http//www.google.com/searchclient=firefox-b-1-d&q=plants+of+family+anacardiaceae.
2. A. Ghani, E. M. Abdurahman, and E. N. Sokomba, "Phytochemical studies on the bark of Sclerocarya birrea (A. Rich.) Hochst," Nigerian Journal of Pharmaceutical Sciences 3, 1 (1987): 33–36.
3. C. A. Uzoho, C. N. Ejezie, and S. I. Ofoefule, "Physco-chemical Properties of Magnifera indica Seed Fat used as Suppository Base," Nigerian Journal of Natural Products & Medicine 1, 1 (1997): 32–34.
4. A. C. Kudi et al., "Screening of some Nigerian medicinal plants for anti-bacterial activity," Journal of Ethnopharmacology 67, 2 (1999): 225–228.
5. J. A. O. Ojewole, "Hypoglycemic effect of Sclerocarya birrea {(A. Rich) Hochst} (Anacardiaceae) Stem-bark Aqueous Extract in Rats," Phytomedicine 10 (2003): 675–681.
6. "Evaluation of the anti-inflammatory properties of Sclerocarya birrea {(A. Rich) Hochst} (family: Anacardiaceae) Stem-bark Extracts in Rats," Journal of Ethnopharmacology 85, 2–3: 217–220.
7. O. Ekungayo, "A review of the volatiles of the Annonaceae," Journal of Essential Oil Research 1 (1989): 223–245.

8. I. T. U. Eshiet, A. Akisanya, and D. A. H. Taylor, "Diterpenes from Annona senegalensis," Phytochemistry 10, 12 (1971): 3294–3295.

9. A. O. Ogundaini, F. O. Ogungbamila, and T. A Olugbade, "Volatile oil from the seed of Mondora myristica, (Dunal)," Journal of the West African Pharmacy 5, 182 (1991): 25–26.

10. A. Adesumoju et al., "Volatile contituents of Monodora tenuifolia fruit oil," Journal of Medicinal Plant Research 57 (1991): 299–398.

11. J. O. Moody, P. J. Hyland, and D. H. Bray, "Bioactive constituents of Enantia chlorantha Oliv," 8th International Symposium on Medicinal Plants (1992): 91.

12. O. Ekundayo et al., "Volatile oil constituents of Dennettia tripetalla," Planta Medica, 58 (1992): 386.

13. O. O. Ebong, B. A. Wariso, and I. Orupabo, "The gastrointestinal inhibitory actions of Xylopia aethiopicum (Dunal) A. Rich (Annonaceae) in rats," West African Journal of Pharmacology and Drug Research 11 (1995): 94–98.

14. E. O. Ajaiyeoba et al., "Synthesis and antifungal activities of 2-phenylnitroethane; a component of Dennetia tripetalla fruits and Nitro vinyl Derivatives," Journal of Pharmaceutical Research and Development 4, 1 (1999): 47–52.

15. Ibid.

16. S. A. Igwe, J. C. Afonne, and S. I. Ghasic, "Ocular dynamics of systemic aqueous extracts of Xylopia aethiopica (African guinea pepper) seeds on visually active volunteers," J of Ethnopharmacol 86, 2–3 (2003): 139–142.

17. O. T. Adeniyi and B. A. Adeniyi, "Antimicrobial and cytotoxic activities of the fruit essential oil of Xylopia aethiopica from Nigeria," Fitoterapia 75, 3–4 (2004): 386–370.

18. K. Boakye-Yiadom, N. Fiagbe, and S. Ayim, "Antimicrobial properties of some West African medicinal plants IV. Antimicrobial activity of Xylopic acid and other constituents of the fruits of Xylopia aethiopica (Annonaceae)," Lloydia 40, 6 (1977): 543–545.

19. M. Iwu, Handbook of African Medicinal Plants (Boca Raton, Florida: CRC Press, 1993).

20. U. A. Utoh-Nedosa, "Evaluation of the Antimicrobial Effects of Ethanol and Water Extract of Dry Fruits of Xylopia aethiopica (Duna) A. Rich on bacterial and fungal isolates," International Conference on Traditional Medicine, Jos.

21. K. Boakye-Yiadom, N. Fiagbe, and S. Ayim, "Antimicrobial properties of some West African medicinal plants IV. Antimicrobial activity of Xylopic acid and other constituents of the fruits of Xylopia aethiopica (Annonaceae)," Lloydia 40, 6 (1977): 543–545.

22. U. A. Utoh-Nedosa, "Evaluation of the Antimicrobial Effects of Ethanol and Water Extract of Dry Fruits of Xylopia aethiopica (Duna) A. Rich on bacterial and fungal isolates," International Conference on Traditional Medicine, Jos.

23. L. N. Tatsadjieu et al., "Antibacterial and antifungal activity of Xylopia aethiopica, Monodora mystica, Zanthoxylum xanthoxyloides and Zanthoxylum leprieuril from Cameroon," Fitoterapia 74, 5 (2003): 469–472.

24. O. T. Adeniyi and B. A. Adeniyi, "Antimicrobial and cytotoxic activities of the fruit essential oil of Xylopia aethiopica from Nigeria," Fitoterapia 75, 3–4 (2004): 386–370.

25. Chrissie S. Abaidoo, Eric Woode, and Abass Alhassan, "An evaluation of the effect of ethanolic fruit extracts of Xylopia aethiopica on haematological and biochemical parameters in male rats," Der Pharmacia Sinca 2, 2 (2011): 39–45.

26. Eze Kingsley Nwangwa, "Anti-fertility effects of ethanolic extract of Xylopia aethiopica on male reproductive organ of Wistar rats," American Journal of Medicine and Medical Sciences 2, 1 (2012): 12–15.

27. Aphrodite T. Choumessi et al., "Cell division," 7, 8 (2012), accessed 1/3/16, http://www.com/content/7/1/8.

CHAPTER 5

Effects of Plants of Family *Caricaceae* and Family *Cucurbitaceae* as Evidenced by Scientific Researches

FAMILY *CARICACEAE* IS made of four genera and fifty-five species of trees found mainly in tropical Africa and America. A well-known example of this family is the partially woody pawpaw or papaya tree whose unripe green fruits provide milky white juice, papain (when incised), which is used in gastrointestinal therapeutics as a "digestive" substance.

Research Studies on Plants of Family *Caricaceae*

Antidiabetic potency of pawpaw (*Carica papaya*) was evaluated in alloxan-induced white albino rats with extract of mature unripe pawpaw fruits using chlorpropamide as the standard positive control. The pawpaw extract lowered blood glucose effectively in a manner comparable to the action of chlorpropamide.

Preliminary phytochemical screening of the pawpaw extract showed that it contained carbohydrates, glucose, amino acids, fixed and volatile oils, and glucosinolate.[1]

The potentials of pawpaw (*Carica papaya*) seeds as a treatment for nematodiasis in village goats were evaluated in nine West African Dwarf goats that were positive for helminthiasis. The goats were randomly divided into three groups to serve for the administration of 5g and 10g milled pawpaw seeds, and the control group was given water. The most prevalent worm detected in the goats was *Haemonchus contortus* (53.9%) followed by *Nematodirus spathiger* (23.2%), *Ostertagia circumcineta* (12.1%), and *Cooperia* spp. (10.8%).

The treatments were given six times at two weeks' interval. Fecal samples were collected for helminth count. Bodyweight changes were recorded and blood parameters were investigated.

The results of the study showed that the pawpaw seed treatment was effective as an anti-helminthic as the 10 g seed powder produced 31.0%–51.4% reduction of the helminth infection in the goats, and the 5 g seed powder produced 28%–48% reduction of the helminth infection in the goats.

The blood parameters monitored, the packed cell volume; the erythrocyte count and hemoglobin concentration, increased with the treatments. These results suggested the potentials of pawpaw (*Carica papaya*) seeds as a treatment for nematodiasis in West African Dwarf goats.[2]

The effect of *Carica papaya* seed extract that contains benzyl isothiocyanates, one of the inducers of phase 11 enzymes in the regulation of stress, was investigated on U937 cells (human monocyte/macrophage cell line). The cellular responses of the U937 cells were observed with the administration of extract concentrations of 200 mg/mL, 500 mg/mL, and 100 mg/mL (ppm) for twenty-four to forty-eight hours.

Results of the study showed that the U937 cells cultured with each of the dose regimens of the *Carica papaya* seed extract had a lower population of apoptotic/transformed cells in a dose-dependent manner with active proliferation of the cells.[3]

Blood pressure depression by the fruit juice of *Carica papaya* (L) in renal and DOCA-induced hypertension in rats, showed that unripe fruits of *Carica papaya* contain antihypertensive principles that possess mainly α-adrenoceptor activity.[4]

A derivative of papain, chymopapain is reported to be sometimes used intravenously in orthopedic surgery to dissolve the nucleus of the intervertebral disc in cases of herniated lumber or trapped nerves.[5] This function of chymopapain, in conjunction with the use of papain as a "digestive enzyme," generated the reference to the papaya tree a "digestive" and a "vermifuge."[6]

The chloroform extract of *Carica papaya* (Linn) seeds decreased the sperm concentration in langur monkeys[7] and high doses (800 mg/kg) of aqueous extract of *Carica papaya* seeds exhibited abortifacient properties on female Sprague-Dawley rats.[8]

The protective effect of dried fruits of *Carica papaya* on hepatotoxicity[9] has also been reported.

Topical application of the juice of unripe fruit of pawpaw promoted dislodging, granulation, and healing; reduced odor in chronic ulcers and was more effective than other topical applications in the treatment of chronic ulcers.[10] Trials were effective in dislodging necrotic tissue and preventing infection of burns.[11]

The latex or sap of *Carica papaya* has antifungal[12] and anti-amoeba properties.[13] The latex of the unripe fruit of pawpaw and crystalline papain produced anti-ulcer effects by significantly reducing histamine-induced acid secretion in chronic gastric fistulated-rats.[14]

Antimicrobial and antioxidant activities of unripe papaya were also demonstrated.[15] The seed and pulp of *Carica papaya* demonstrated antibacterial activities against many organisms like *Escherichia coli*, *Enterobacter cloacae*, *Bacillus subtillis*, and *Salmonella typhi*; and the same seed and pulp of the plant showed antioxidant activity comparable to those of soybean paste miso, rice bran, and baker's yeast.[16]

Research Studies on Plants of Family *Cucurbitaceae*

Results of in vivo administration of *Momordica charantia* extracts in Sprague-Dawley rats showed that the extract caused an increase in muscle and liver protein levels but produced a decrease in brain protein and a decrease in muscle and liver glycogen. The extract also caused a decrease in the activities of serum L-alanine transaminase and alkaline phosphatase but caused a slight elevation of the levels of serum alkaline aspartate transaminase and adenosine triphosphatase activities.

The ethanol extract of *Momordica charantia* did not affect the level of the activity of L-aspartate transaminase but decreased the activity of adenosine triphosphatase.[17] These results suggest that *Momordica charantia* extracts act by inhibition of adenosine triphosphatase activity, which amounts to inhibition of the energy metabolism of the organ or organism.

An investigation of the modulatory effect of *Momordica charantia* extract on the plasma and intestinal Ca^{2+} ATPase in normal and alloxan-induced diabetic rabbits showed that the extract of the plant, significantly ($P < 0.05$) reduced the fasting blood sugar levels of both normal and diabetic rats by 37.69% and 145.8% respectively within eight weeks of treatment thus confirming the hypoglycaemic properties of *Momordica charantia*.

It was also observed that during the period of execution of the hypoglycaemic activity, the *Momordica charantia* extract increased the activity of erythrocyte Ca^{2+} ATPase in the alloxan-induced diabetic rabbits by 67.57%, but the extract did not affect the activity of erythrocyte Ca^{2+} ATPase in the control rabbits. Also, the basal activity of erythrocyte Ca^{2+} ATPase in the alloxan-induced diabetic rabbits was reduced by 87.5% by the extract when it did not affect the activity of erythrocyte Ca^{2+} ATPase in the control rabbits.[18]

The activity of the calcium pump of the intestinal mucosa of the extract-treated alloxan-induced diabetic rabbits was slightly higher than those of controls.[19]

These results suggested that the hypoglycaemic activity of *Momordica charantia* extract modulates the activity of the Ca^{2+} pumping ATPase in diabetics.

Edible oil was mechanically extracted from *Citrullus colocynthis* (guna melon) seed and characterized.

Results of the study showed that 54.7%±0.82% of the oil was from the kernel, and 43.3 ± 0.60% of the oil was from the unshelled seed by weight. The moisture content, free fatty acid content, iodine value, saponification value, and unsaponifiable matter content were 0.13 ± 0.04%, 0.65 ± 0.10%, 109 ± 1.50%, 213.8 ± 4.85%, and 1.05 ± 0.06% respectively. The fatty acid composition determined by gas-liquid chromatography (GLC) showed the individual unsaturated fatty acids to be oleic acid (18.1), 15.5 ± 0.07%; linoleic acid (18.2), 15.69 ± 1.04%; and linolenic acid (18.3), 15.01 ± 0.02%. The composition of the unsaturated fatty acids was palmitic acid (16.0), 10.3 ± 0.42%, and stearic acid (18.0), 14.7 ± 0.68%. The unidentified fatty acids constituted 2.5 ± 0.04%.[20]

Chromatographic and spectroscopic analysis of bound and unbound phenolic acids in *Lagenaria breviflora a Cucurbitaceae* fruit used in Nigerian folk medicine as an antibacterial and an antifertility drug, showed that p-hydroxybenzoic and vanillic acids occurred as free and bound acids in the pulp while ferulic acid occurred only as an ester. Isolation and characterization of these compounds were done with column chromatography (TLC, PC, UV, IR, and GC-MS) techniques.[21]

Three new saponins were isolated from the fruit pulp of *Lagenaria breviflora*. The saponins were characterized as 3-O-β-galactopyranosyl, 28-O-β-xylopyranosyl-(1-4)-α-rhamnopyranosyl(1-3)-β-xylopyranosyl(1-

3)-α-arabinopyrosylolean-12-en-28-oic acid ester, 3-O-β-galactopyrano-28-O-β-galactopyranosyl(1-4)-α-rhamnopyranosyl(1-3)-β-xylopyranosyl(1-3)-α-arabinopyrosylolean-12-oic acid ester, and 3-O-β-galactopyranosyl-28-O-β-arabinopyranosyl(1-6)-β-galactopyranosyl(1-4)-α-rhamnopyranosyl(1-3)-xylopyranosyl(1-3)-α-arabinopyranosylolean-12-en-28-oic acid ester.

Oleanolic acid and 3-O-acetyloleanolic acid were isolated from the hydrolytic products of *Lagenaria breviflora* fruit pulp.[20]

Hypoglycaemic action of *Momordica charantia* extracts was demonstrated in human subjects[22] and validated in an animal model of diabetes.[23] An insulin-like constituent found in *Mormordica charantia* seed extracts[24] thought to account for the hypoglycaemic effects of these extracts was extracted.[25] An isolate, "Charantin" was found to be more potent than tolbutamide in hypoglycaemic activity.[26] A similar active hypoglycaemic compound foetidin was extracted from a related plant, *Momordica foetida*.[27]

Abortifacient effects were observed in extracts of the roots of *Momordica augustisepala*.[28] Oxycitocic activity and antiimplantation activity was exhibited by extract of the fruit of *Lagenaria breviflora*.[29], [30], [31], [32] The extracts of both plants of the family *Cucurbitaceae* are employed in folk medicine as antifertility phytomedicines.

The aqueous extract of the fruit of *Legenaria brevifolia* elicited potent oxytocic effect on isolated uterine strips of pregnant and nonpregnant rats. The methanol extract of the fruit showed 60%, 70%, and 90% abortifacient activity for early-trimester, midtrimester, and late-trimester pregnancy in eight-week pregnant albino rats at a dose of 0.65g/kg per day for three days.

A dose of 2.0 g/kg, 2.5 g/kg, and 5 g/kg methanol extract of the *Legenaria brevifolia* fruit gave 60%, 80%, and 100% anti-implantation activity, respectively.

Phytochemical screening showed traces of cardiac glycosides in the seed of plants of family *Cucurbitaceae*. It also showed that saponins, tannins, fixed oils, mucilage reducing sugars and carbohydrates are present in the fruit of plants of this family. There is usually the absence of alkaloids, cyanogenic glycosides, and cucurbitacins.[33]

References

1. J. M. Oke, "Anti-diabetic potency of pawpaw, Carica papaya," African Journal of Biomedical Research 1 (1998): 31–34.
2. M. A. Dipeolu, D. Eruvbetine, and M. O. Abiola, "Potentials of pawpaw (Carica papaya) seeds as treatment for nematodiasis in village goats," The Bioprospector 1, 1 (1999): 15–20.
3. O. Dosumu et al., "Carica papaya extract enhances cellular response to stress in U937," Nigerian Journal of Health and Biomedical Sciences 2, 2 (2003): 94–97.
4. A. E. Eno et al., "Blood pressure depression by the fruit juice of Carica papaya (L) in renal and DOCA-induced hypertension in rats," Phytotherapy Research 14, 4 (2000): 235–239.
5. "Papaya: Carica papaya L," Purdue University, http://www.hort.purdue.edu/newcrop/morton/papaya ars.html.
6. G. D. Pamplona-Roger, "Papaya Tree-Digestive and Vermifuge," in Encyclopaedia of Medicinal Plants: Education and Health Library (Toledo, Spain: Artes Graficas, 1998), 1435.
7. N. K. Lohiya et al., "Chloroform extract of Carica papaya induces long-term reversible azoospermia in langur monkey," Asian J Androl 4 (2002): 17–26.

8. O. Oderinde et al., "Abortifacient properties of aqueous extract of Carica papaya (linn) seeds on female Sprague-Dawley rats," Nier Postgraduate Med. J. 9, 2 (2002): 95–98.

9. B. Rajikapoor et al., "Effect of dried fruits of Carica papaya on hepatotoxicity," Biol Pharm Bull 12 (2002): 1645–1646.

10. H. Hewitt et al., "Topical use of Papaya in chronic skin ulcer therapy in Jamaica," West Indian Med. J. 49, 1 (2000): 32–33.

11. I. F. Starley et al., "The treatment of paediatric Burns using topical papaya," Burns 25, 7s (1999): 36–39.

12. H. Hewitt et al., "Topical use of Papaya in chronic skin ulcer therapy in Jamaica," West Indian Med. J. 49, 1 (2000): 32–33.

13. I. F. Starley et al., "The treatment of paediatric Burns using topical papaya," Burns 25, 7s (1999): 36–39.

14. R. Giordani et al., "Fungicidal activity of latex sap from Carica papaya and anti-fungal effect of D-(+)-glucosamine on Candida albicans, Mycoses 39, 3–4 (1996): 103–110.

15. L. Tona, K. Kambu, and N. Njimbi, "Anti-amoebic and phytochemical screening of some Congolese medicinal plants," J. Ethnopharmacol 61, 1 (1998): 57–65.

16. Ibid.

17. C. F. Chen et al., "Protective effects of Carica papaya Linn on the exogenous gastric ulcer in rats," Am J Chin Med 9, 3 (1981): 205–212.

18. J. A. Osato et al., "Antimicrobial and antioxidant activities of unripe papaya," Life Sci. 53, 17 (1993): 1383–1389.

19. O. O. Oyedapo and B. G. Araba, "Stimulation of protein biosynthesis in rat hepatocytes by extracts of Momordica charantia," Phytotherapy Research 15 (2001): 95–98.

20. T. O. Bamidele et al., "The modulatory effect of Momordica charantia on the plasma and intestinal Ca2+ ATPase in normal and alloxan-induced diabetic rabbits," Nigerian Journal of Pharmaceutical Research 1, 1 (2002): 26.

21. M. O. Oresanya et al., "Extraction and characterization of Citrullus colocynthis seed oil," Nigerian Journal of Natural Products and Medicine 4 (2000): 76–78.

22. A. A. Elujoba, A. F. Fell, and A. Linley, "Chromatographic and Spectroscopic Analysis of Bound and unbound Phenolic acids in Lagenaria breviflora fruit," Journal of Pharmaceutical and Biomedical Analysis 9, 9 (1991): 711–715.

23. A. A. Elujoba et al., "Triterpenoids from the fruit of Lagenaria breviflora," Phytochemistry 29, 10 (1990): 3281–3285.

24. J. Welihinda et al., "Effect of Momordica charantia on the glucose tolerance in maturity onset diabetes," J. Ethnopharmacol 17, 3 (1986): 277–282.

25. S. Sarkar, M. Pranava, and R. Marita, "Demonstration of the hypoglycaemic action of Momordica charantia in validated animal model of diabetes," Pharmacol Research 33 (1996): 1–4.

26. T. B. Ng et al., "Insulin-like molecules in Momordica charantia seeds," J. Ethnopharmacol 15 (1986): 107–117.

27. P. Khanna et al., "Extraction of insulin from a plant source," 3rd International Congress on Plant Tissue and Cell Cultures (July 21–26, 1974), Leicester, UK.

28. "What is bitter melon (Momordica charantia): What is bitter melon used for today?" M. Derrida, http://www.mdidea.com/products/herbextract/bittermelon/data.html.

29. A. A. Olaniyi, "Chemical investigation of medicinal plants in Nigeria: the isolation of 'Foetidin', from Momordica foetida (Schum and Thorn)," 2nd OAU/STRC Inter-African Symposium on Traditional Pharmacopoeia and African Medicinal Plants (1975).

30. C. N. Aguwa and G. C. Mittal, "Abortifacient effects of the roots of Momordica augustisepala," Journal of Ethnopharmacology 7, 2 (1983): 169–173.

31. A. U. Ogan, "An oxytocic extractive from a West African cucurbit: studies on West African Medicinal Plants-8," Planta Medica 21, 4 (1972): 431–434.

32. J. A. O. Ojewole and A. A. Elujoba, "Preliminary investigation of the oxytocic action of an aqueous extract of Lagenaria breviflora fruit," International Journal of Crude Drug Research 20, 4 (1982): 157–163.

33. A. U. Ogan, "An oxytocic extractive from a West African cucurbit: studies on West African Medicinal Plants-8," Planta Medica 21, 4 (1972): 431–434.

CHAPTER 6

Effects of Medicinal Plants of Family *Leguminosae* as Evidenced by Scientific Research Studies on Their Extracts and Juices

Plants of Family *Leguminosae*

FAMILY *LEGUMINOSAE* CONTAINS six hundred genera and twelve thousand species.[1] Its subfamilies include *Papilionaceae*, *Caesalpinaceae*, and *Mimosaceae* (Mimosoideae). Examples of plants of this family include *Crotolaria* spp., natal indigo, groundnuts, pigeon pea, cowpea, soybeans, Calabar bean, senna species, cassia species, and lentils.

Subfamily Papillionaceae

Plants of this subfamily include *Crotalaria, Indigofera, Astralagus, Mucuna, Erythrina, Phaseolus, Arachis, Abrus, Glycine, Sophora*, and *Trigonella* species.[2] Products obtained from trees of this family include licorice root; Calabar bean; tonco seed; fenugreek seed; tolu balsam; Peru balsam, tragacanth gum; derris, Arachis oil; *Lonchocarpus*; soy oil, cake and milk; copaiba; oleoresin; copals and indigo. Many of these are used as food, drinks, and drugs.

Subfamily Caesalpinaceae

Members of this subfamily of leguminous plants are trees and shrubs examples of which are cassia species: *Cassia occidentalis, Cassia alata, Cassia podocarpa, Cassia tora, Cassia siamea, Cassia fistula, Cassia siebriana, Cassia acutifolia* (senna), *Cassia nigrans, Cassia spectabilis*, and redwood.

Products obtained from plants of subfamily Caesalpinaceae include tamarinds; senna pods and leaves; cassia pods; sassy bark and carob beans.

Subfamily Mimosaceae (Mimosoideae)

Trees of this subfamily of *Leguminosae* are small plants or trees whose fruits are pods. The leaves of many mimosa trees give a tactile response of simultaneous shutting inwards of its leaflets at the slightest tactile pressure including pressure from the air that emerged from the mouth of a person giving a command to a small mimosa tree of six inches above the ground to close its leaves, from a standing position. When I was four to six years old my playmates and I enjoyed standing for several minutes at a time watching small mimosa plants obey our commands, which we issued to them from standing position, 'to open or close their crown of leaf-stalks and leaflets'. Examples of mimosa trees are acacia species.

Products obtained from trees of this subfamily are acacia gum from acacia species; volatile oils like oil of Cassie from acacia species and wattle barks used in tanning obtained from acacia species.

Research Findings on Plants of Family *Leguminosae*

Leaf extracts of *Indigofera arrecta* demonstrated antidiabetic activity in normoglycaemic and streptozoto-cin-induced diabetic rats. Also, diabetic patients given three daily doses of aqueous leaf extract of *Indigofera arrecta* family *Papilionaceae*, after meals, showed significant improvement in their condition. Their fasting blood glucose levels dropped from 250mg/dl to 120mg/dl in three months. Safety evaluation of the *Indigofera arrecta* extract was done in non-diabetic human volunteers.[3] The basis for the antiglycaemic activity of *Indigofera arrecta* extract was evaluated in rats.[2]

Hot aqueous extract of *Indigofera arrecta* exhibited anti-ulcerogenic activity in vivo and in human trials.[4]

The diterpene ent-16a-hydroxykauran-18-oic acid was isolated from the extract of leaves of *Piliostigma thonningii*.[5]

C-methylflavonoids from the leaves of *Piliostigma thonningii* were tested for their ability to inhibit prostaglandin synthesis and antibacterial activity against *Staphlococcus aureus*. These compounds were C-methylflavonoids; 6,8-di-C-methylquercetin 3-methyl ether; 6-C-methylquercetin 3,7-dimethyl ether; quercetin; quercitrin; 6,8-di-C-methyl-kempferol 3-methylether; and 6,8-di-C-methyl kempferol 3,7-dimethyl ether. The study found that the C-methylflavonoids exhibited antibacterial activity and inhibited prostaglandin synthesis and these activities were influenced by the presence of the β ring 3', 4'-diol group.[6]

Chemical and spectroscopic analysis of the volatile oils obtained from the leaves of *Cassia alata* (Caesalpinaceae and Rubiaceae) indicated the presence of the following compounds: sesquiterpene hydrocarbons, sesquiterpene lactones, phenolic compounds, and aromatic polycarboxylic acids.[7]

The methanol extract of the fruit of *Tetrapleura tetraptera* (Mimosaceae) killed the snail *Bulinus globosus* in a concentration of 1ppm–3ppm in twenty-four hours. The methanol extract was eleven times as active as the water extract in this molluscicidal activity. All parts of the plant possessed molluscicidal activity with no phytotoxicity and multiple treatments killed the juvenile and adult snails.[8]

In another study, water extract of *Tetrapleura tetraptera* demonstrated high efficacy in the control of the snail *Biomphalaria glabrata* at a concentration of 24 mg/L in selected water contact sites for twenty-four months.[9]

At a concentration of 7.5-60 mg/L, the water extract of *Tetrapleura tetraptera* caused a dose and time-dependent slowing of the heart of intact *Biomphalaria glabrata*.[10]

Scopoletin (7-hydroxy-6-methoxycoumarin), was isolated from powdered *Tetrapleura tetraptera* (Mimosaceae) by high-performance TLC-spectrofluorimetry at 325nm and by photography.[11] On the other hand, the fruit pulp of the same plant yielded aridanin (a 3-O-[β-D-glucopyranosyl-2'-acetamido-deoxy]-oleanolic acid) as well as hentriacontane, phenylpropanoids, and carbohydrates.[12]

Investigation of the mechanism of the hypotensive effect of scopoletin showed that scopoletin inhibited the indirect electrical stimulation-evoked contractions of the cat nictating membrane in vivo and also inhibited the contractions of isolated perfused central ear artery of rabbit induced by electrical stimulation or by intraluminal noradrenaline administration. Scopoletin also: (1) inhibited the spontaneous, myogenic pendular, rhythmic contractions of the rabbit isolated duodenum; (2) attenuated the indirect electrical stimulation-provoked by exogenous nor-adrenaline contractions of the muscle preparation; and (3) depressed the electrical stimulation-evoked contractions of the chick isolated esophagus. These results in which scopoletin relaxed all the smooth muscles examined suggest that Sscopoletin produced hypotension by smooth muscle relaxant action on the blood vessels.[13]

Volatile oil extracted from the fresh fruits of *Tetrapleura tetraptera*, given intraperitoneally, offered some protection against leptazol-induced convulsions. A dose of 0.4 mL of the oil per mouse, protected 78% of the tested mice from the convulsions when administered thirty minutes before administration of leptazol. Although 0.6 mL did not stop unprotected mice from death as a result of convulsions, it prolonged the onset of convulsions and the time of death.[14]

Similarly, intraperitoneally administered aqueous root and stem extracts of *Cilliandra portoricensis* (family Mimosaceae) demonstrated anticonvulsant activity in pentylenetetrazole and electric shock-induced convulsions in mice.[15]

Low concentrations of Aridanin (0.125 ppm, 0.25 ppm, 0.5 ppm, and 1.0 ppm) and low concentrations of standard molluscicide niclosamide (0.025 ppm, 0.05 ppm, and 0.10 ppm) caused a significant reduction of the egg production of *Biomphalaria glabrata* and *Lymanaea columella*, suggesting that low concentrations of aridanin can produce effective molluscicidal action if released with speed.[16]

Chronic application of sublethal concentrations of aridanin isolated from *Tetrapleura tetraptera* (0.25-0.125 ppm) and of Bayluscide, a standard molluscicide (0.05-0.025 ppm), on *Biomphalaria glabrata* produced significant reductions in the glycogen of the snails while a significant decrease in the protein content of the snails did not occur until after four weeks of continuous exposure, suggesting that aridanin and Vayluscide produce molluscicidal action on the carbohydrate metabolism of the snail.[17]

Methysergide and cyproheptadine antagonized the contractions produced by serotonin. Verapamil, lanthanum, and cyproheptadine inhibited the actions of aridanin, suggesting a calcium-dependent action of aridanin and serotonin receptor as the site of action of aridanin on gut tissue.[18]

Aridan, a water extract of *Tetrapleura tetraptera* and aridanin (a glycoside isolated from the fruit of the same plant), did not affect cell proliferation and did not induce chromosomal aberrations or affect sister chromatid exchanges in Chinese hamster ovary cells cultured in vitro. The two substances, aridan and aridanin, did not also show mutagenic activity in *Salmonella typhimurium* strains TA 97, TA 98, and TA 100 in the presence or absence of a metabolizing system. These results suggest that the use of aridan or aridanin is not likely to produce genotoxicity.[19]

Water and ethanol extract of *Daniella oliveri* exhibited antimicrobial activity against standard *E. coli* NCTC10418 and clinical isolates (*Staph aureus, Proteus mirabilis, Pseudomonas aeruginosa, Klebsiella* spp., and *E. coli*). The water extract of *Daniella oliveri* was more potent in antimicrobial activity than the ethanol extract which showed no antimicrobial activity at low doses.[20]

The stem bark extract of *Daniella oliveri* exhibited antagonism of histamine-induced contractions of guinea pig ileum and noncompetitive inhibition of acetylcholine-induced contractions of the frog rectus abdominis muscle,[21] which suggest the production of its activity by interaction with serotonin receptors.[22]

Metabolic cage studies with stem bark extract of *Daniella oliveri* showed that a 70% alcohol extract of this stem bark caused a significant decrease in body weight, food intake, and urine and stool output.[23]

Hexane, ethylacetate, and methanol fractions of stem bark extract of *Daniella oliveri* were tested for analgesic, antipyretic, and anti-inflammatory activities. The hexane extract fraction exhibited analgesic activity while the methanol extract fraction exhibited anti-inflammatory activity; and the ethyl acetate fraction was inactive in the induced analgesia, pyretic, and inflammatory conditions tested.[24]

The flavonoid 7-4'-dimethoxy-2-hydroxyformononetin, an isoflavone, was isolated from the heartwood of *Pycanthus angolensis* (Mimosaceae) while the flavonoids sativan and medicarpin were isolated from the heartwood of *Baphia nitida* (Mimosaceae).[25]

A study determined the physical and emulsifying properties of the powdered, aqueous, and methanol extracts of the fruit of *Tetrapleura tetraptera* and compared them with those of *Quillaia tincture* BP.

The equilibrum surface tension of the extracts was achieved after twelve hours. Emulsions prepared with liquid paraffin, cod liver oil, and peppermint oil as oil phases resulted in a hydrophile-lipophile balance of 10, 11.25, and 11.25 respectively for the aqueous extract, powdered extract, and the *Quillaia tincture*. The aqueous extract formed the best emulsion but none of the extracts formed micelles in water.

The droplet size of the emulsions decreased with increasing concentrations of the extracts and increased with storage.[26]

The flavonoid-rich fraction of the leaf of *Baphia nitida* obtained by a chromatographic process was formulated into an ointment and tested at three dose levels for anti-inflammatory activity against croton oil and heat-induced inflammation on ears of mice and depilated backs of rats. Hydrocortisyl cream was used as the positive control of the experiment.

The flavonoid-rich fraction of *Baphia nitida* leaf extract produced a dose-related anti-inflammatory response by inhibiting the inflammation of the mice and rats. The mouse ear model was more sensitive than the rat back model. Hydrocortisyl cream was significantly active in both the mice and rat models.[27]

Phytochemical and pharmacological studies on stem bark of *Detarium microcarpum* Guill. and Perr. (*Leguminosae*) revealed that the extract contained cardiac and saponin glycosides and condensed tannins.

In comparison with a standard antipyretic and analgesic drug, acetylsalicylic acid, the stem bark extract of *Detarium microcarpum* demonstrated dose-related antipyretic and analgesic activity.[28]

The root extract of *Cilliandra portoricensis* (family Mimosaceae) produced sustained and dose-dependent contractions of guinea pig ileum, which was compared to those of acetylcholine and histamine on the same tissue. The relative order of agonist potency (EC_{50}) was 3.5×10^{-3} mg > 2.8×10^{-2} mg > 4.17 mg for acetyl-choline (ACh), histamine, and *Cilliandra portoricensis* extract (CPE) respectively.

Atropine (60×10^{-11} – 1.2×10^{-9} M) competitively blocked CPE-induced contractions (PA_2 = 9.2, 0.04; slope = 1.1 ± 0.02). Higher atropine concentrations produced noncompetitive block of these contractions.

Pirezepine (3.2×10^{-9} – 2.16×10^{-8} M) shifted the dose-response curve to the right (PA_2 = 7.82, 0'08; slope = 1.4 ± 0.2) while mepyramine (2.5×10^{-9} – 2.5×10^{-9} M) did not affect the CPE-induced contractions.[26] The competitive block of CPE contractions by low dose atropine (60×10^{-11} – 1.2×10^{-9} M), no block by mepyramine, and noncompetitive block of CPE contractions by higher doses of atropine suggest that CPE produced its contractions at α subunits of serotonin receptors of guinea pig ileum.[29]

Physical and chemical analysis of *Voandzeia subterranean* (Bambara nut) determined through proximate analysis showed *Voandzeia subterranean* peas contain 9.7% moisture, 16.6% protein, 5.9% fat, 2.9% ash, 4.9% crude fiber, and 64.9% carbohydrate.

Maximum water absorption of *Voandzeia subterranean* peas was attained after soaking for eleven, nine, six, and four hours at 25°C, 40°C, 50°C, and 60°C, respectively. Maximum dehauling efficiency of the Bambara nut seeds was obtained when the seed absorbed 54.7% water at 60°C and dried for nine hours.

The study of the microstructure of the seed and raw flour of the seed showed that they contained starch granules and proteins of different sizes.

Milling disorganized the arrangements of the starch granules and protein units while cooking the flour paste caused all the components of the Bambara seed flour to lose their identity and intergrity.[30]

The following compounds were isolated and identified from *Philostigma thonningii* by spectral methods especially 2D-NMR: philostigmiin, a 2-phenoxychromone; 6-8-di-methylquercetin 3,7-dimethyl ether; 6-C-methylquercetin 3,7-dimethyl ether; 6,8-di-C-methylquercetin 3,7-dimethyl ether; quercetin; quercitrin, 6-C-methylquercetin 3-methyl ether; 6,8-di-C-methylkaempferol 3,7-dimethyl ether; 6,8-di-C-methylkaempferol 3-methyl ether; and 6,8-di-C-methylkempferol 3,7-dimethyl ether28.

A study was made regarding the antimicrobial activity and preliminary phytochemical screening of the seed of *Mucuna pruriens* against typed strains of *Staphylococcus aureus*, *Escherichia coli*, *Pseudomonas aeruginosa*, *Klebsiella pneumonia*, *Salmonella gallinorum*, *Bacillus subtilis* NCTC 6571, and clinical isolates of staphylococcal species and *Proteus mirabillis* using agar well-diffusion method. The results of the study showed that the seed extract of *Mucuna pruriens* exhibited antimicrobial activity against all organisms tested and that the antimicrobial activity of the extract was highest against *Salmonella gallinarium*.[31]

The molluscicidal activity of extracts of the fruit and leaves of Dialium *guineense* were found to be attributable to oleanolic acid saponins, three of which were isolated from the fruit and a fourth of which was isolated from the leaves of the plant.[32]

Studies were done on the seed oils of *Parkia biglobosa* and *Parkia bicolor* by gas chromatography (GC) and gas chromatography-mass spectrometropy (GC-MS) techniques to determine their fatty acid composition. The results showed that the seed oils of *Parkia bicolor* contained six major fatty acids and that the seed oils of *Parkia biglobosa* contained five major fatty acids.

The seed oils of both *Parkia biglobosa* and *Parkia bicolor* contained five similar fatty acids in almost the same ratios. Arachidic acid was the most abundant fatty acid being greater than 40% in both oils.

The other fatty acids in the oils were stearic, behenic, palmitic, and linoleic acids. The sixth fatty acid in *Parkia bicolor* seed oil was an unsaturated fatty acid called bicolargic acid ($C_{20}H_{3}7COOH$). The study also found that the seed oils of *Parkia biglobosa* and *Parkia bicolor* were nontoxic.[33]

Subchronic experiments were conducted with low concentrations of saponins from *Tetrapleura tetraptera* (Mimosaceae) and Bayluscide to study the ultrastructural effects of these molluscicides on *Biomphalaria glabrata*.

The results of the study showed that (1) the ratio of the digestive cells of the snail to the crypt cells was inverted in the molluscicide-treated snails and (2) dose-dependent autolytic areas were also observed in the small foot connective tissues of the molluscicide-treated snails.[34]

The major ultrastructural effects of the molluscicides were seen in the digestive gland of the molluscicide-treated snails. These effects consisted of dose-dependent autolysis of the membrane structures of organelles like the mitochondria; the Golgi apparatus and the endoplasmic reticulum.[35]

These results suggest that the *Tetrapleura tetraptera* and Bayluscide molluscicides bring about the death of treated *Biomphalaria glabrata* snails by (1) inhibiting their energy metabolism and organelles like the mitochondria, thereby causing autolysis of membrane structures of important organelles like rough endoplasmic reticular where protein synthesis takes place. Dose-dependent autolytic areas observed in the small foot connective tissues of the molluscicide-treated snails suggest that the small foot of the treated snails had become progressively destroyed, thereby blocking the movement of the snails to find food. Autolysis of membrane structures of digestive glands of the treated snails will eventually block digestive activity resulting in the death of the snails by their ingested food not being digested.

The extractable constituents of the bark of *Calliandra haematocephala* (Mimosaceae), fractionated by chromatographic techniques, produced the following compounds: p-hydroxybenzoic acid, caffeic acid, protocatechuic acid, astilbin, neoisoastilbin, and catechin-3-O-rhamnoside. These isolated compounds showed varying antibacterial activities. Lupeol and betulinic acid were isolated from the nonactive fraction of the extract.[36]

Phytochemical and antibacterial properties of *Parkia biglobosa* and *Parkia bicolor* (Mimosaceae) leaf extracts showed that the hexane, ethyl acetate, water, and ethanol extracts of both plants exhibited similar concentration-dependent antimicrobial activities and inhibited the growth of gram-positive bacteria, though the extracts of *Parkia bicolor* showed slightly higher antimicrobial activity than those of *Parkia biglobosa*. The organisms used in the study included *Staphylococcus aureus*, *Bacillus cereus*, *Pseudomonas aeruginosa*, *Escherichia coli*, *Aspergillus niger*, and *Candida utilis*.[37]

Cassia occidentalis (Caesalpinaceae) was found to have laxative, abortifacient, cholagogic, diuretic, and tonic properties.[38] Some studies have also found that *Cassia occidentalis* has antimalarial properties[39] and exerted protective effects against chromosomal aberrations in mice.[40]

Cassia occidentalis was also shown to contain anthraquinone glycosides,[41] which could have contributed to toxic cardiomyopathy observed in biochemical studies in *Cassia occidentalis*-poisoned rabbits.[42]

The dried leaves of *Cassia podocarpa* (Caesalpinaceae) have been shown to possess laxative and purgative properties.[4344] The anthraquinone content of *Cassia podocarpa* was less than that of the official senna. Aqueous infusion and methanol extract of *Cassia podocarpa* showed in vitro antidiarrheal effect.[45] The concentration of the *Cassia podocarpa* extract and the prevailing gastrointestinal environment seem to determine the direction of activity of the extract (whether the extract would be purgative or antidiarrheal).

A multicentre randomized controlled trial of *Cassia alata* Linn for constipation found that its leaf infusions administered at bedtime have stronger purgative action compared to placebo. The study also found that 16%–25% of the participants reported minor side effects like nausea, dyspepsia, abdominal pain, and diarrhea.[46]

Ethanol extracts of *Cassia alata* exhibited high fungicidal activity against dermatophytic fungi but low activity against other fungal forms.[47, 48]

Cassia alata leaf extract exhibited high analgesic activity compared to kaempferol 3-O-sophoroside in a study in which morphine was used as the positive control.[49]

Flavonoid glycosides were isolated from *Cassia alata* extracts.[50]

In vitro antimalarial activity of leaf extracts of *Cassia occidentalis* and *Guiera senegalensis* on *Plasmodium yoelii nigerensis* showed that malarial parasite growth was completely inhibited by 100 μg/mL and 1,000 μg/mL of the extract; chloroquine (6 μg/mL) was used as the positive control for the experiment.[51] Another evaluation in vivo and in vitro of antimalarial activity of two leaf extracts of *Cassia occidentalis* showed that the two extracts exhibited high prophylactic but low suppressive (antimalarial) activity.[52]

Chemical analysis showed the major constituent of *Cajanus cajan* (soya bean) seeds to be an amino glycoside and hydroxycinnamic acid.[53] Chemical analysis also showed the major constituent of the protein of these seeds to be a large number of aromatic amino acids which have been reported in some studies to possess antisickling properties.[54]

Chemical evaluation of the nutrient and tannin composition of fermented oil bean, castor oil bean, and African locust bean used as food condiments of Nigeria (fermented for varying periods) showed that the four-day fermentation period caused the highest increases in protein and tannin and the highest decreases in ash, lipids, and nonprotein nitrogen. The pulp of African locust bean had more protein and ash while the oil bean seeds had fewer lipids and nonprotein nitrogen.

Fermentation for four days increased zinc, sodium, and phosphorus for the African locust bean; but its pulp had lower zinc and phosphorus than the seed. The study showed that the four-day fermentation period was the best for the production of nutrients by fermented oil bean, castor oil bean, and African locust bean used as food condiments in Nigeria.[55]

Preliminary study on the antimicrobial activities of *Cassia tora* and *Cassia occidentalis* on *E. coli*, *P. aerugenosa*, *Staph. aureus*, and *Candida albicans* showed that antimicrobial activity of diethyl/ethanol, water, and methanol extracts was better than that of chloroform extract. The minimum inhibitory concentration of *Cassia tora* extracts against the organisms was 1.56-12.5 mg/mL while the MIC for *Cassia occidentalis* was 25-100 mg/mL.[56]

Antibacterial evaluations of *Cassia alata* leaf extract showed that it had broad-spectrum activity against two-gram-positive bacteria (*Staphycoconcus aureus* NCTC 6571 and *Bacillis subtillis* NCTC 8236) and two-gram-negative bacteria (*Escherichia coli* NCTC 10418 and *Pseudomonas aeruginosa* ATCC 10145). The antibacterial activity of the extract was comparable to that of streptomycin sulfate (1 mg/mL) used as the standard drug.[57]

Laxative properties of cassia pods sourced from Nigeria—*Cassia alata* LC, *Cassia hirsuta*, *Cassia occidentalis* LC, *Cassia podocarpa* Guill. and Perr., *Cassia siamea* Lam, *Cassia fistula*, *Cassia acutifolia*, and *Cassia siebriana* L (family Caesalpinoidae or Caesalpinaceae)—were evaluated with white albino rats with *Cassia acutifolia* Del. (senna) pod tablet and leaf as reference standard drugs.

Infusions of the pods of *Cassia podocarpa*, *Cassia fistula*, and *Cassia acutifolia* and the leaf of *Cassia acutifolia* at a dose range of 100 mg/kg to 700mg/kg produced wet feces in tested rats, which was an indication of laxative action. Statistical analysis of variance and using percentage senna-pod action showed that the laxative potencies of the infusions of the pods of Cassia *podocarpa*, *Cassia fistula*, and *Cassia acutifolia* were not significantly different from those of senna-pod infusions.[58]

Infusions of the pods of *Cassia podocarpa*, *Cassia fistula*, and *Cassia spectabilis* exhibited higher antifungal activity than those of their leaf samples. Their pod extracts showed good antibacterial activity when compared with the effects of ampicillin.[59]

Seasonal variations of hydroxyanthraquinone content were shown to occur in cultivated *Cassia spectabilis* leaves. Concentrations of hydroxyanthraquinone (1.03%) significantly ($P < 0.05$) peaked in the leaves during the dry season (September to January) and significantly decreased in the leaves during the rainy season.[60]

Seasonal accumulation of anthraquinones was also observed in leaves of cultivated *Cassia podocarpa*. Combined anthraquinones concentrated (2.43%) in the leaves at peak flowering and were lowest in the bark (0.21%). Anthraquinone glycosides reached peak levels between October and March and reached the highest levels between January and March. On the other hand, there was a drop in anthraquinone glycosides between April and September which is the rainy season period in Nigeria.

The concentration of aglycones in the plant samples increased slightly during the rainy season period, which is favorable for the laxative activity and reduced toxicity of these plant extracts.[61]

Acute toxicity and phytochemical studies of graded doses of aqueous extract of *Cassia occidentalis* in rats showed that LD_{50} of the extract was 1,680 mg/kg body weight. Dose-dependent mortality occurred in rats given 1,200 mg/kg, 1,800 mg/kg, and 3,200 mg/kg.

Phytochemical studies of the *Cassia occidentalis* extract showed that it contained tannins, anthraquinones, sterols, saponins, glycosides, and alkaloids.[62]

Evaluation of the antifungal property of the aqueous and ethanol crude extracts of the bark of *Brachystegia eurycoma* and the leaves of *Richardia brasilensis* using agar disc-diffusion method showed that after forty-eight hours of incubation, 2 mg/mL dose of these four extracts inhibited the growth of *Aspergilius niger*, *Aspergilius flavus*, *Aspergilius fumigatus*, *Candida albicans*, *Epidermophyton floccosium*, *Fusarium solani*, *Microsporium audonii*, *Trichophyton verrucosum*, and *Mucor mucedo*.

The ethanol extract of the leaves of *Richardia brasilensis* was the most active of the four extracts. On the other hand, the water extracts of the bark of *Brachystegia eurycoma* was more active than its ethanol extract.

Preliminary phytochemical studies showed that the water extract of the leaves of *Richardia brasilensis* contained mainly tannins while its ethanol extract contained anthraquinone, saponins, flavonoids, phlobatanin, and steroids. The aqueous extract of the bark of *Brachystegia eurycoma* contained mainly tannin while its ethanol extract had flavonoids and tannins. Alkaloids and terpenes were absent in the four examined extracts.[63]

The anti-nociceptive and smooth muscle contracting activities of methanol extract of *Cassia tora* leaf were evaluated. The extract (LD_{50} in mice, > 2,000 mg/kg, i.p., and p.o.) contracted smooth muscles of guinea pig ileum and rabbit jejunum in a concentration-dependent manner, which was blocked by atropine. The extract also increased intestinal transit time in a concentration-dependent manner.

The extract also significantly ($P < 0.05$), reduced the number of acetic acid-induced abdominal constrictions in mice with an effect that was comparable with those of aspirin (150 mg/kg i.p.) and also dose-dependently significantly ($P < 0.05$) reduced the nociceptive response of mice to increased force (g).[64]

These results authenticated the folk use of extracts of *Cassia tora* as a laxative and for the treatment of intestinal colic.

Water extracts of fresh young leaves and fresh mature leaves of *Cassia alata* collected at 0600, 1200, and 1800 hours were tested undiluted (100%) and as 50%, 25%, and 12.5% dilutions, fresh and after two days' storage on *Candida pseudotropicalis* NCYC for antifungal activity. The antifungal activity of the freshly made and two days-stored aqueous extracts of fresh, young, and old leaves of *Cassia alata* demonstrated antifungal activity comparable to that of acriflavine (6 mg/mL) used as the positive control.[65]

Three C-methylflavonoids; 6-C-methylquercetin-3; 3C,4C-trimethyl ether; 6-C-methylkaempferol-3-methyl ether; 6,8-di-C-methylkaempferol-3-7-dimethyl ether and piliostigmin (2-phenoxychrome); quercetin; quercetirin; and quercetin-3-O-glucoside were isolated from the leaves of *Piilostigma reticulatum*.[66]

The methanol extract and fractions of *Cassia nigrans* Vahl (*Caesalpinacea*) used in Central Nigeria for the treatment of ulcer and intestinal ailments were evaluated for antimicrobial activity and their effects on *Helicobacter pylori*. The extract (2,000 mg/mL) was tested against *Candida*, *Pseudomonas*, *Bacillus*, *Salmonella*,

Shigella, Klebsiella species, and *Helicobacter pylori*. The MIC of the crude methanol extract and three fractions against *Helicobacter* was 125 mg/mL to 200 mg/mL and against the other organisms were 550 mg/mL, 1,050 mg/mL, 300 mg/mL, and 260 mg/mL to 500 mg/mL. The high activity of the methanol extract and fractions of *Cassia nigrans* against the tested organisms justified its folk use for intestinal disorders.[67]

Pharmacological investigations were done on in vivo laxative activity in rats; effects on isolated guinea pig ileum and toxicological screening of an aqueous infusion of the pods of *Cassia fistula*. The results of the study showed that the extract of the pods produced a potent dose-dependent laxative activity between 100 mg/kg and 500 mg/kg per ounce in rats. The extract also produced a dose-dependent inhibition of the normal rhythmic contraction of the isolated guinea pig ileum at concentrations of 4 mg/mL to 8 mg/mL, which was not blocked by the adrenergic receptor antagonist, phentolamine, at a concentration of 10^{-8} M. The calculated LD value of the extract was 6.6 g /kg per ounce.

The subclinical, clinical, and histopathological findings on the liver, kidney, and testis of the *Cassia fistula* pod-extract-treated rats did not show any differences between control and treated rats. These results suggest the efficacy and safety of Cassia fistula pods as a laxative drug.[68]

Other studies on plants of family *Leguminosae* that can be consulted for further reading include the following:

1. Evaluation of the antidiarrhoeal activity of the methanolic/methylene (50:50) extract of the leaves of *Desmodium velitinum* (fam. Fabaceae).[69]
2. Antipyretic and phytochemical evaluation of the ethanol extract of the leaves of *Desmodium velutinum*.[70]
3. Increment on the quality protein fraction of cooked *Voandzeia subterranean* (hypogeal) seed flour paste meal by added soya beans (*Glycean max*) and cowpea (*Vigna unguinata*) portions.[71]
4. Dependence of particle size, texture, protein content, and shelf life of *Voandzeia hypogea* bean cakes on flour paste preparation-water temperature.[72]
5. An investigation into the ulcer activity of the methanol extract of *Stemonocoleus micranthus* Harms bark (family Leguminoseae).[73]
6. An investigation into the antipyretic activity of n-hexane extract of the leaves of *Baphia pubescens*.[74]
7. Anti-inflammatory, phytochemical, and toxicological investigations of ethanol extract of the leaves of *Baphia pubescens* Hook F (family *Leguminosae*).[75]
8. An investigation into the anti-inflammatory activity of n-hexane extract of the leaves of *Baphia pubescens* Hook F (family *Leguminosae*).[76]
9. Analgesic, phytochemical, and toxicological investigations of ethanol extract of the leaves of *Baphia pubescens* Hook (family *Leguminosae*).[77]
10. Antipyretic, phytochemical, and toxicological investigations of ethanol extract of the leaves of *Baphia pubescens* Hook F (family *Leguminosae*).[78]

References

1. Charles Evans, Trease and Evans Pharmacognosy, 16th ed. (Edinburgh: Saunders, 2009).
2. Ibid.
3. A. A. Sittie and A. K. Nyako, "Indigofera arrecta: safety evaluation of an anti-diabetic plant extract in non-diabetic human volunteers," Phytother Res. 12, 1 (1998): 52–54.

4. "Anti-ulcerogenic activity of hot aqueous extract of powdered Indigofera affecta, in vivo," Wambebe (2000), www.sciweb.com/features/patents/patents.

5. M. T. Martin et al., "Complete 1H and 13C NMR assignment of a Kaurane Diterpene from Piliostigma thonningii," Magnetic Resonance in Chemistry 35 (1997): 896–898.

6. J. C. Ibewuike et al., "Anti-inflammatory and anti-bacterial activities of C-methylflavonoids from Piliostigma thonningii" (1997).

7. T. V. Benjamine, "Phytochemical and Biological analysis of some local anti-eczematic plants," 4th OAU/STRC Inter-Africa Symposium on Traditional Pharmacopoeia African Medicinal Plants (1979): 493–495.

8. C. O. Adewunmi, S. K. Adesina, and V. O. Marquis, "The laboratory and field evaluation of the molluscicidal properties of Tetrapleura tetraptera" (1982).

9. C. O. Adewunmi, "Water extract of Tetrapleura tetraptera: an effective molluscicide for the control of Schistosomiasis and Fascioliasis in Nigeria," Journal of Animal Production and Research 4, 1 (1984): 73–84.

10. Ibid.

11. E. E. Essien, S. K. Adesina, and J. Reisch, "Quantitative analysis of Scopoletin in the fruit of Tetrapleura tetraptera Taub. (Mimosaceae)," Scientia Pharmacetica 51 (1983): 397–402.

12. S. K. Adesina and J. Reisch, "A triterpenoid glycoside from Tetrapleura tetraptera fruit," Phytochemistry 24, 12 (1985): 3003–3006.

13. J. A. Ojewale and S. K. Adesina, "Mechanism of the hypotensive effect of Scopoletin isolated from the fruit of Tetrapleura tetraptera, Planta. Medica 49 (1983): 46–50.

14. J. I. Nwaiwu and P. A. Akah, "Anticonvulsant effect of the volatile oil from the fruit of Tetrapleura tetraptera," Journal of Ethnopharmacology 18, 2 (1986): 103–107.

15. P. A. Akah and J. I. Nwaiwu, "Anticonvulsant activity of root and stem extracts of Calliandra portoricensis," Journal of Ethnopharmacology 22, 2 (1988): 205–210.

16. C. O. Adewunmi, P. Furu, and H. Madsen, "Evaluation of the effects of low concentrations of Aridanin isolated from Tetrapleura tetraptera Taub. (Mimosaceae), on the growth and egg production of Biomphalaria glabrata and Lymanaea columella Say," Phytotherapy Research 3, 3 (1989): 81–84.

17. Ibid.

18. C. O. Adewunmi, G. Dorfler, and W. Becker, "Effect of Aridanin isolated from Tetrapleura tetraptera and serotonin on the isolated gastrointestinal tract smooth muscle of Biomphalaria glabrata and uptake of calcium," Journal of Natural Products 53 (1990): 956–959.

19. C. O. Adewunmi, H. C. Anderson, and L. Busk, "A potential molluscicide, Aridan (Tetrapleura tetraptera), neither induces chromosomal alteration in Chinese Hamster Ovary Cells nor mutations in Salmonella typhimurium," Toxicology and Environmental Chemistry 30 (1991): 69–74.

20. S. Ntiejumokwu and D. N. Onwukaeme, "Antimicrobial and Preliminary Phytochemical Screening of the Leaves of Daniella oliveri (Rolfe) Hutch and Dalz (Leguminosae)," West African Journal of Pharmacology and Drug Research 9, 10 (1991): 95–99.

21. N. D. Onwukaeme, "Pharmacological activities of extracts of Daniella oliveri (Rolfe) Hutch and Dalz (Leguminosae)," Phytotherapy Research 9 (1995): 306–308.

22. Uchechukwu Anastasia Utoh-Nedosa, "Evidence that Adrenergic; Muscarinic; Histaminic; Anti-malarial drugs; Opioid; NSAID, Nicotinic; Vasodilator drugs; Rauwolfian alkaloid and Adenosine Receptors are Parts or Whole of the Serotonin Receptor: chick rectum studies," Track 3, International Summit on Clinical Pharmacy and Dispensing, Hilton San Antonio Airport Hotel, Texas, USA (November 2013): 18–20.

23. N. D. Onwukaeme, "Pharmacological activities of extracts of Daniella oliveri (Rolfe) Hutch and Dalz (Leguminosae)," Phytotherapy Research 9 (1995): 306–308.

24. Ibid.

25. O. R. Omobuwajo, S. A. Adesanya, and G. O. Babalola, "Isoflavonoids from Pycnanthus angolensis and Baphia nitida," Phytochemistry 31, 3 (1992): 1013–1014.

26. L. O. Orafidiya, O. O. Faniran, and J. I. Olaifa, "Physical and emulsifying properties of the fruit extracts of Tetrapleura tetraptera (Schum and Thonn) Taub. (Mimosaceae)" (1994).

27. N. D. Onwukaeme, "Anti-inflammatory activities of flavonoids of Baphia nitida Lodd. (Leguminosae), on mice and rats," Journal of Ethnopharmacology 46, 2 (1995): 121–124.

28. N. D. Onwukaeme, "Phytochemical and Pharmacological studies on Stem Bark of Detarium microcarpum (Guill. & Perr.) (Leguminosae)," Journal of West African Pharmacology 9 (1995): 1.

29. Ibid.

30. N. J. Enwere and Y. C. Hung, "Some chemical and physical properties of Bambara groundnut, (Voandzeia subterranean Thours) seed and products," International Journal of Food Science & Nutrition 47, 6 (1996): 469–75.

31. J. C. Aguiyi et al., "Antimicrobial activity and preliminary phytochemical screening of the seed of Mucuna pruriens, (Linn) DC," West African Journal of Biological Sciences 5, 1 (1996): 71–76.

32. O. A. Odukoya et al., "Molluscicidal triterpenoid glycosides of Dialium guineense," Journal of Natural Products 59 (1996): 632–634.

33. A. A. Aiyelaagbe, E. O. Ajaiyeoba, and O. Ekundayo, "Studies on the seed oils of Parkia biglobosa and Parkia bicolor," Plant Foods for Human Nutrition 49 (1996): 229–233.

34. A. U. D. Bode et al., "The effects of extracts from Tetrapleura tetraptera (Taub.) and Bayluscide on cells and tissue structures of Biomphalaria glabrata (Say.)," Journal of Ethnopharmacology 50 (1996): 103–113.

35. Ibid.

36. R. Nia et al., "Adesina Antibacterial Constituents of Calliandra haematocepala," Nigerian Journal of Natural Products and Medicine 3 (1999): 58–60.

37. E. Ajaiyeoba, "Phytochemical and anti-bacterial properties of Parkia biglobosa and Parkia bicolor (Mimosaceae) leaf extracts," African Journal of Biomedical Research 5 (2002): 125–129.

38. A. L. Ake, "Some medicinal properties of Cassia occidentalis, Caesalpinaceae, in the lower Ivory Coast," Bothalia 14 (1983): 617–620.

39. L. Tona et al., "In vivo antimalarial activity of Cassia occidentalis, Morinda morindoides and Phyllantus niruri," Drug Chem. Toxicol 22 (1999): 643–53.

40. N. Sharma et al., "Protective effect of Cassia occidentalis extract on chemical-induced chromosomal aberrations in mice," Ann. Trop. Med. And Parasitol. 95, 1 (2001): 47–57.

41. P. P. Rai and M. Shok, "Anthraquinone glycosides from plants of Cassia occidentalis," Indian J. Chem. 45 (1983): 87–88.

42. P. J. O'Hara and K. R. Pierce, "Toxic cardiomyopathy caused by Cassia occidentalis, 11 Biochemical studies in poisoned rabbits," Vet. Pathol. 11 (1974): 110–124.

43. S. O. Larbi and R. A. Lewis, "Biological assay of Cassia podocarpa: a plant related to senna," West African J. Pharmacol Drug Res. 3, 2 (1976): 149–152.

44. A. A. Akiremi, O. R. Omobuwayo, and A. A. Elujoba, "Pharmacopoeial standards for the fruits of Cassia fistula and Cassia Podocarpa," Nigerian J. Nat. Prodand Med. 4 (2000): 23–26.

45. R. O. Akomolafe et al., "An In vitro study of the effects of Cassia podocarpa fruit on the intestinal motility of rats," Phytomed 11, 2–3 (2004): 249–54.

46. V. Tamlikitkul et al., "Randomised controlled trial of Cassia alata Linn. for constipation," J. Med Assoc. Thai 73, 4 (1990): 217–22.

47. S. Palanichamy, "Antifungal activity of Cassia alata leaf extract," J. Ethnopharmacol 29, 3 (1990): 337–340.

48. S. Damodaran and S. Venkataraman, "A study on the therapeutic efficacy of Cassia alata leaf extract against Pityriasis versicolor," J. Ethnopharmacol 42, 1 (1994): 19–23.

49. S. Palanichamy and S. J. Nagarajan, "Analgesic activity of Cassia alata leaf extract and kaempferol-3-O-sophoroside," Ethnopharmacol 29, 1 (1990): 73–8.

50. D. Gupta, "Flavonoid glycosides from Cassia alata," Phytochem. 30, 8 (1991): 2761–2763.

51. E. O. Iwalewa et al., "In vitro anti-malarial activity of leaf extracts of Cassia occidentalis and Guiera senegalensis on Plassmodium yoelii nigerensis," West African Journal of Pharmacology and Drug Research 4 (1990): 19–21.

52. B. E. Akinde, I. Okeke, and O. O. Orafidiya, "Phytochemical and anti-bacterial evaluations of Cassia alata leaf extract," West African Journal of Pharmacy 13, 1 (1999): 36–40.

53. J. O. Onah, M. M Iwu, and P. I. Akubue, "Part structure elucidation of some chemical constituents of aqueous fraction of Cajanus cajan seeds," West African Journal of Pharmacology and Drug Research 9, 10 (1991): 127.

54. J. O. Onah, M. M Iwu, and P. I. Akubue, "The chemistry of glycoproteins (Cajanin), isolated from the seeds of Cajanus cajan," West African Journal of Pharmacology and Drug Research 9, 10 (1991): 126.

55. I. C. Obizoba and L. N. Atu, "Production and chemical evaluation of some food condiments of Nigeria," Plant Foods and Human Nutrition 44, 3 (1993): 249–254.

56. J. A Onaolapo, P. P. Rai, and E. N. Sokomba, "Preliminary study on the antimicrobial activities of Cassia tora and Cassia occidentalis," Glimpsies in Plant Research 11 (1993): 533–536.

57. B. E. Akinde, I. Okeke, and O. O. Orafidiya, "Phytochemical and anti-bacterial evaluations of Cassia alata leaf extract," West African Journal of Pharmacy 13, 1 (1999): 36–40.

58. A. A. Elujoba, A. T. Abere, and S. A. Adelusi, "Laxative properties of Cassia pods sourced from Nigeria," Nigerian Journal of Natural Products & Medicine 3 (1999): 51–53.

59. K. A. Abo, S. W. Lasaki, and A. A. Adeyemi, "Laxative and anti-microbial properties of Cassia species growing in Ibadan," Nigerian Journal of Natural Products & Medicine 3 (1999): 47–50.

60. K. A. Abo et al., "Seasonal variations of hydroxyanthraquinone content of cultivated Cassia spectabilis," African Journal of medicine and Medical Science 29, 2 (2000): 141–144.

61. K. A. Abo and A. A. Adeyemi, "Seasonal accumulation of anthraquinones in leaves of cultivated Cassia podocarpa Guill. et Perr.," African Journal of Medicine and Medical Science 31, 2 (2002): 171–173.

62. S. A. Muyibi et al., "Acute toxicity and phytochemical studies of Cassia occidentalis Linn. extract in rats," Journal of Veterinary Science 2, 2 (2000): 22–25.

63. A. A. Adekunle, "Antifungal property of the crude extract of Brachystegia eurycoma and Richardia brasilensis," Nigerian Journal of Natural Products and Medicine 4 (2000): 70–72.

64. F. C. Chidume et al., "Anti-nociceptive and smooth muscle contracting activities of methanol extract of Cassia tora leaf," Journal of Ethnopharmacology 81, 2 (2002): 205–209.

65. K. A. Abo and A. A. Adeyemi, "Seasonal accumulation of anthraquinones in leaves of cultivated Cassia podocarpa Guill. et Perr.," African Journal of Medicine and Medical Science 31, 2 (2002): 171–173.

66. B. E. Akinde, O. O. Oradifaya, and A. O. Oyedele, "The effect of time of collection and storage on the antifungal activity of fresh Cassia alata Linn (Caesalpinaceae) aqueous leaf extract from old and young leaves," Nigerian Journal of Pharmaceutical Research 1, 1 (2002): 95–96.

67. O. Obiageri et al., "Antimicrobial screening of extracts and fractions of Cassia nigrans Vahl (Caesalpinacea) and their effects on Helicobacter pylori," Nigerian Journal of Natural Products and Medicine 7 (2003): 82.

68. M. A. Akanmu et al., "Pharmacological investigations and toxicological screening of an aqueous infusion of the pods of Cassia fistula in rodents," African Journal of Biomedical Research 6, 3 (2003).

69. C. F. Anowi et al., "Evaluation of antidiarrhoeal activity of the methanolic/methylene (50:50) of the leaves of Desmodium velitinum Fam Fabaceae," IJPI's Journal of Pharmacognosy and Herbal Formulations, www.ijpijournals.com.

70. Anowi Chinedu Fred, Onyegbule Ahamefule Felix, Onyekaba Theophilus, Azode Chinwe, "Antipyretic and phytochemical evaluation of the ethanol extract of the leaves of Desmodium velutinum," Asian Journal of Pharmacy and Life Sciences 2, 2 (2012): 340–345.

71. Uchechukwu Utoh-Nedosa, Nedosa Ikenna Valentine, Anowi Chinedu Fred, "Increment on the quality protein fraction of cooked Voandzeia subterranean (hypogeal) seed flour paste meal by added Soya beans (Glycean max) and cow pea (Vigna unguinata) portions," Herald Journal of Agriculture and Food Science Research 2, 2 (2013): 82–85.

72. Uchechukwu Anastasia Utoh-Nedosa, Nedosa Ikenna Valentine, Anowi Chinedu Fred, "Dependance of particle size, texture, protein content and shelf life of Voandzeia hypogea bean cakes on flour taste preparation-water temperature," Herald Journal of Agriculture and Food Sciences Research 2, 4 (2013): 117–122.

73. C. C. Ezea et al., "Investigation into the ulcer activity of the methanol extract of Stemonocoleus micranthus Harms bark (fam Leguminoseae)," World Journal of Pharmaceutical Research 3, 3 (2014): 3669–3675.

74. Anowi Chinedu Fred et al., "An investigation into the antipyretic activity of n-hexane extract of the leaves of Baphia pubescens. Hook F. Family Leguminosae," JPP (Journal of Pharmacognosy and Phytochemistry) 3, 2 (2014): 127–131.

75. Anowi Chinedu Fredrick et al., "Anti-inflammatory, phytochemical and toxicological investigations of ethanol extract of the leaves of Baphia Pubescens Hook F (family Leguminosae)," AJBPR (Asian Journal of Biochemical and Pharmaceutical Research) 2, 4 (2014).

76. Anowi Chinedu Fredrick et al., "An investigation into the anti-inflammatory activity of n-hexane extract of the leaves of Baphia pubescens Hook F (family Leguminosae)," JPCBS (Journal of Pharmaceutical, Chemical and Biological Sciences) 2, 2 (2014).

77. Anowi Chinedu Fredrick et al., "Analgesic, phyochemical and toxicological investigations of ethanol extract of the leaves of Baphia pubescens Hook, Family Leguminosae," Universal Journal of Pharmacy 3, 4 (2014):11–16.

78. Anowi Chinedu Fredrick et al., "Antipyretic, phytochemical and toxicological investigations of ethanol extract of the leaves of Baphia pubescens Hook. F (Family: Leguminosae)," IJPPR (International Journal of Pharmaceutical and Phytopharmacological Research) 5, 2 (2015): 1–8.

CHAPTER 7

The Effects of Medicinal Plants of Family *Compositae* and Family *Asteraceae* as Evidenced by Scientific Researches on Them

Family *Compositae*

FAMILY *COMPOSITAE* CONTAINS about nine hundred genera and thirteen thousand species.[1] Plants of *Compositae* family usually have large numbers of tiny flowers or florets arranged in heads in copious panicles. Examples of plants of family *Compositae* are *Vernonia* spp., *Zinnia* spp., artemisia, chrysanthemum, *Carduus*, dahlia, *Ageratum conzoides*, sunflower, etc. Plants of family *Asteraceae* are often included among the plants of family Compsitae.

Some Scientific Researches on Plants of *Compositae* and *Asteraceae* Families

The effects of chloroform, methanol, and aqueous extracts of powdered leaves of *Vernonia amygdalina* (*Asteraceae*) and *Eupatorium odoratum* (Euphorbiaceae) on blood clotting time were evaluated using a liver method and whole blood clotting time method. The effects of these extracts were compared with those of controls (distilled water for the aqueous extract and 96% alcohol for the chloroform and methanol extracts) because the extracts were dissolved in 96% alcohol for use in the test.

The results of the study showed that the aqueous and methanol extracts had anticoagulant activity, but the chloroform extract did not have this activity. None of the three extracts exhibited hemostatic activity. Phytochemical screening of the methanol and chloroform extracts showed that the methanol extract indicated the presence of saponins and tannins while the chloroform extract indicated the presence of terpenes and steroids.[2]

The effect of four test fractions of ethanol extract of powdered leaves of *Vernonia amygdalina* on the rate of gastric emptying was evaluated in rats. The rate of gastric emptying of a test meal was evaluated one hour after the feeding of the rat.

The results of the study showed that each of the four test fractions reduced the rate of gastric emptying in the tested rats which did not occur in the control rats.[3]

The dose-related blood sugar-lowering effect of *Vernonia amygdalina* (*Asteraceae*) was demonstrated by its aqueous leaf extract in a rabbit model. A dose of 80 mg/kg body weight produced a maximum lowering of blood sugar level of both fasted normal and fasted alloxinized rabbits. The fasting blood sugar of normoglycaemic rabbits was reduced from 96 mg% to 48 mg% in four hours and the fasting blood sugar of the alloxinized rabbits was reduced from the mean value of 520 mg% to 300 mg% in eight hours. The LD_{50} of *Vernonia amygdalina* extract given by intraperitoneal injection in mice was 1,122 mg/kg body weight, indicating that administration of 1.1 gram per body weight to the animal was safe.[4]

The pharmacological effects of dichloromethanol extract of *Inula crithmoides* L (*Compositae*) were evaluated in vivo and in vitro. The extract showed low acute toxicity; dose-dependently decreased arterial blood pressure and manifested analgesic, anti-inflammatory, and central nervous system-depressor activity.

Preincubation of guinea pig ileum and rat duodenum with the extract greatly reduced the contractile effect of histamine and acetylcholine on these tissues and produced a dose-related inhibition of the effects of serotonin. The ethylene chloride/acetone (50/50) fraction of the extract reduced the threshold of chemically stimulated pain and produced a great decrease in motor activity.[5] These results show that pharmacological effects of dichloromethanol extract from *Inula crithmoides* are mainly inhibitory and are produced at serotonin receptors because of the dose-related inhibition of the effects of exogenous serotonin.

Aqueous, dichloromethane, and methanol extracts of *Helichrysum aureonitens* (*Asteraceae*), were evaluated for antibacterial activity against five-gram-positive and five-gram-negative organisms. The dichloromethane extract was active against five of the gram-positive organisms. The methanol extract was active against three of the gram-positive organisms while the aqueous extract was not active against any of the organisms. The dichloromethane and methanol extracts were not active against the gram-negative bacteria.[6]

A study evaluated the antiviral activity of crude aqueous extracts of shoots of *Helichrysum aureonitens* (*Asteraceae*) against herpes simplex virus type 1 (HSV-1) in vitro.

At a concentration of 1.35 mg/mL (w/v) of the aqueous extract of shoots of *Helichrysum aureonitens* showed strong inhibition of herpes simplex virus type 1 in human lung fibroblasts as demonstrated by the absence of a cytopathic effect.[7]

Hydroxytremetone was isolated from the flowers of *Tagetes patula* (*Asteraceae*) and was also detected in extracts of the leaf and stem of the plant.[8]

Evaluation of the carthartic effect of the leaf extract of *Vernonia amygdalina* in mice showed that that the extract showed a strong promotion of intestinal motility on charcoal meal test in mice. The frequency of defecation and feces discharge was markedly increased following administration of the extract.

The leaf extract of *Vernonia amygdalina* also promoted gastric emptying in rats and produced a contractile effect on isolated rat fundus which was blocked by atropine.[9]

Aqueous and methanol extracts of *Emilia sonchifolia* leaves were evaluated for anti-inflammatory properties on rat paw edema induced by subplantar injection of albumin. The study found that both aqueous and methanol extracts of *Emilia sonchifolia* leaves progressively reduced rat paw edema and thus had anti-inflammatory properties. The aqueous extract of *Emilia sonchifolia* leaves produced more pronounced anti-inflammatory effects than the methanol extract.[10]

The toxicological effects of chronic administration of water extracts of leaves of *Ageratum conyzoides* were investigated in rats.

The results of the study showed that the LD_{50} of the extract was 600 mg/kg. Post mortem changes that are associated with acute toxicity of the extract included generalized congestion of the liver, kidney, and intestines and petechial hemorrhages along the intestinal tract and on the subcutaneous muscles. Paracentral hepatic necrosis was also observed.[11]

Toxicological histopathological changes observed on termination of chronic administration of the extract were dose-dependent lesions observed in sections of the liver, kidney, and intestines.[12]

Medicinal application of *Vernonia amygdalina* Del leaf in treatment of schistosomiasis in mice was studied by testing the effect of petroleum ether and ethanol extracts of *Vernonia amygdalina* on mice infected with a two-hundred-dose *Schistosoma mansoni* type cercariae obtained from *Biomphalaria pfeifferi* snails by intraperitoneal inoculation. The petroleum ether extract or the ethanol extract of *Vernonia amygdalina* leaf extract were given by intraperitoneal injection to the infected animals at a dose of 1 mg/kg body weight for five consecutive days following the detection of lateral spined eggs (ten weeks post-inoculation) in their feces. One group of infected untreated mice served as the positive control, one group that was not infected served as the negative control, while another group that served as the test for prophylactic action of the extract, received a single prophylactic dose of 1 mg/kg body weight twenty-four hours before inoculation of the animals.

Prophylactic application of the extracts recorded 34.06% and there was reduction of parasite load by petroleum ether extract and ethanol extract respectively. The infected untreated group was anemic with enlarged and congested liver, spleen, and kidney, with necrotized areas and severe enteritis; while the negative controls showed no adverse histopathological changes. The petroleum ether extract and the ethanol extract reduced the parasite load by 83.61% and 72.3% respectively.[13] These results suggest that *Vernonia amygdalina* leaf extract has prophylactic and curative effects on the causative agent of schistosomiasis.

Anti-inflammatory and antinociceptive effects of the extract of the shoot of *Sphaeranthus senegalensis* (*Asteraceae*) (used in folk medicine for the treatment of rheumatism and other ailments) was evaluated in mice and rats against egg albumen-induced rat hind paw edema; acetic acid-induced abdominal constriction; hot plate test in mice; and the formalin pain test in rats. Saline was used as the test compound for the control animals.

The results showed that the *Sphaeranthus senegalensis* extract produced significant ($P < 0.05$) dose-dependent anti-inflammatory and anti-nociceptive effects in all test models examined thereby authenticating the folk medicinal use of the plant,[14] for pain and inflammatory conditions.

Similarly, the anti-inflammatory, analgesic, and antipyretic effects of 100 mg/mL, 200 mg/mL, and 400 mg/mL intraperitoneal injections of methanol, chloroform, and ether extracts of the leaves of *Vernonia cinerea* (*Asteraceae*) were evaluated with acetic acid-induced writhing in mice; carrageenan-induced rat paw edema and brewer's yeast-induced pyrexia in rats.

The results showed that the extracts significantly (P < 0.05) inhibited the acetic acid-induced writhing in mice; reduced the pyrexia and paw volumes in rats and increased the pain threshold in the oedematous hind limb of rats. These results demonstrated that *Vernonia cinerea* leaf extract possesses anti-inflammatory, analgesic, and antipyretic properties;[15] and these properties may be responsible for the use of the plant in traditional Nigerian medicine for the treatment of malaria.

The effect of aqueous extract and fractions of aqueous leaf extract of *Vernonia amygdalina* on human breast cancer cell DNA synthesis was evaluated on MCF cell line considered a suitable model for this evaluation.

Treatment of MCF cell line with concentrations of a water-soluble extract of *Vernonia amygdalina* and fractions of the extract produced a potent dose-dependent inhibition of DNA synthesis of MCF cells both in the presence and absence of serum. These results suggest that incorporation of *Vernonia amygdalina* vegetable in the diet may prevent or delay the onset of breast cancer.[16]

Ethanol extract of the aerial parts of *Tithonia diversifolia* (*Asteraceae*) and of the stem bark of *Crossopteryx febrifuga* (Rubiaceae) were evaluated on their activity on early, residual, and established malaria on Swiss albino mice in vivo at a dose range of 50-400 mg/kg per day using chloroquine as the positive control drug for the residual infection test.

The extracts gave dose-dependent chemo-suppression at different levels of the infection tested. The suppression of parasitemia by the highest doses of extracts of both *Tithonia diversifolia* (*Asteraceae*) and *Crossopteryx febrifuga* was similar to that of chloroquine and pyrimethamine.

Both ethanol extracts of *Tithonia diversifolia* and *Crossopteryx febrifuga* gave some level of suppression of the early and established phases of the infection. The 200 mg/kg ethanol extract of *Tithonia diversifolia* actively suppressed parasitemia in the residual or repository stage but showed low activity in the suppression of the established infection as the mean survival period of the mice treated with the extract in the established infection test was low. *Crossopteryx febrifuga* extract was inactive in the repository (residual infection) test.[17]

Extracts of *Emila sonchifolia* leaves produced a dose-dependent reduction in blood glucose in dithizone diabetic rats that were of the same pattern as that of the hypoglycaemic drug chlorpropamide.[18]

Studies on *Vernonia amygdalina* demonstrated that extracts of the plant have

- organ (liver)-protective properties;[19, 20, 21, 22]
- antioxidant properties;[23, 24, 25]
- anti-diabetic or hypoglycaemic properties;[26, 27, 28, 29, 30]
- lipid-lowering and anti-obesity properties;[31, 32, 33]
- hemolytic and anticoagulant properties;[34, 35, 36]
- inhibitory, body-stabilizing/body-calming, and sleep-producing properties;[37, 38, 39, 40, 41]
- insect antifeedant, schistosomacidal, and antileishmania properties;[42, 43]
- cathartic properties;[44]
- antimicrobial properties;[45] and
- anticancer/anti-tumor properties.[46, 47, 48, 49]

Vernonia amygdalina demonstrated analgesic, antiplasmodial and anti-malarial properties[50], [51] while another species of *Vernonia* (*Vernonia cinerea*) demonstrated a combination of antipyretic, analgesic, and anti-inflammatory properties, all of which are very important in relieving both malaria and the basic symptoms of most illnesses, which are fever, pain, and inflammation.

References

1. M. D. Barrachina, R. Bello, and J. Esplugues, "Pharmacological evaluation of dichloromethanol extract from Inula crithmoides L," Phythotherapy Research 9 (1995): 294–298.
2. A. C. Igboechi and D. C. Anuforo, "Anticoagulant activities of extracts of Eupatorium odoratum and Vernonia amygdalina," The State of Medicinal Plant Research in Nigeria (1986): 313–320.
3. D. C. Anuforo and A. C. Igboechi, "The effect of Vernonia amygdalina, extracts on gastric emptying time in rats," The State of Medicinal Plant Research in Nigeria (1986): 321–331.
4. P. A. Akah and C. L. Okafor, "Blood sugar lowering effect of Vernonia amygdalina Del. in an experimental rabbit model," Phytotherapy Research 6 (1992): 171–173.
5. M. D. Barrachina, R. Bello, and J. Esplugues, "Pharmacological evaluation of dichloromethanol extract from Inula crithmoides L," Phythotherapy Research 9 (1995): 294–298.
6. J. J. M. Meyer and A. J. Afolayan, "Antibacterial activity of Helichrysum aureonitens (Asteraceae)," Journal of Ethnopharmacology 47, 2 (1995): 109–111.
7. J. J. M. Meyer et al., "Inhibition of herpes simplex virus type 1 by aqueous extracts from shoots of Helichrysum aureonitens (Asteraceae)," Journal of Ethnopharmacology 52, 1 (1996): 41–43.
8. A. J. Ekpo, T. W. Cole Jr., and M. B Polk, "Hydroxytremetone from Tagetes patula," Nigerian Journal of Natural Products and Medicine 2 (1998): 59–60.
9. S. O. Awe, J. M. Makinde, and O. A. Olajide, "Carthatic effect of the leaf of Vernonia amygdalina," Fitoterapia 70 (1999): 161–165.
10. K. N. Muko and F. C. Ohiri, "A preliminary study on the anti-inflammatory properties of Emilia sonchifolia leaf extracts," Fitoterapia 71 (2000): 65–68.
11. B. M. Agaie, P. Nwatsok, and M. L. Sonfada, "Toxicological effects of water extracts of Ageratum conyzoides in rats," Journal of Veterinary Science 2, 2 (2000): 27–31.
12. Ibid.
13. A. U. Ugboli et al., "Medicinal application of Vernonia amygdalina Del leaf in treatment of Schistosomiasis in Mice," Nigerian Journal of Natural Products and Medicine 4 (2000): 73–75.
14. B. Adzu et al., "Anti-inflammatory and anti-nociceptive effects of Sphaeranthus senegalensis," Journal of Ethnopharmacology 84, 2–3 (2003): 169–173.
15. E. O. Iwalewa, O. J. Iwalewa, and J. O. Adeboye, "Analgesic, anti-pyretic and anti-inflammatory effects of methanol, chloroform and ether extracts of Vernonia cinerea Less leaf," Journal of Ethnopharmacology 86 (2003): 229–234.
16. E. B. Izevbigie, "Discovery of water-soluble anticancer agents (edotides) from a vegetable found in Benin City, Nigeria," Experimental Biology and Medicines 228, 3 (2003): 293–298.
17. T. O. Elufioye and J. M. Agbedahusi, "Antimalarial activities of Tithonia diversifolia (Asteraceae) and Crossopteryx febrifuga (Rubiaceae) on mice in vivo," Journal of Ethnopharmacology 31, 57 (2004): 1–5.
18. C. C. Monago and P. A. Ogbomeh, "Anti-diabetic effect of Emila sonchifolia in Dithizone-diabetic rats," Global Journal of Pure and Applied Sciences 10, 1 (2004): 183–187.
19. Adaramoye Oluwatosin, Bayo Ogungbenro, and Anyaegbu Oluchi, "Protective Effects of Extracts of Vernonia amygdalina, Hibiscus sabdariffa and Vitamin C against radiation-induced liver damage in rats," Journal of Radiation Research 49, no. 2 (2008): 123–131.
20. B. A. Iwalokun et al., "Hepatoprotective and Antioxidant Activity of Vernonia amygdalina on Acetoaminophen-Induced Hepatic Damage in Mice," Journal of Medicinal Food 9, 4 (2006): 524–530.
21. Adaramoye Oluwatosin, Bayo Ogungbenro, and Anyaegbu Oluchi, "Protective Effects of Extracts of Vernonia amygdalina, Hibiscus sabdariffa and Vitamin C against radiation-induced liver Damage in Rats," Journal of Radiation Research 49, 2 (2008): 123–131.
22. E. M. Arhoghro et al., "Effect of Aqueous Extract of Bitter Leaf Vernonia amygdalina (Del) on Carbon Tetrachloride (CCl4)-induced Liver Damage in Albino Rats," European Journal of Scientific Research 26, no. 1 (2009): 122–130.

23. Mbang Owolabi et al., "Evaluation of the Antioxidant Activity of the leaves of Vernonia amygdalina," Journal of Complementary and Integrative Medicine 5, 1 (2008).

24. H. U. Nwanjo, "Efficacy of Aqueous Leaf Extract of Vernonia amygdalina on Plasma Lipoprotein and Oxidative Status in Diabetic Rat Models," Nigerian J. of Physiological Sc. 20, 1 (2005).

25. Gregory Avwiri and F. O. Igho, "Inhibitive Action of Vernonia amygdalina on the Acidic Corrosion of (2S and 3RS) Aluminium Alloys in Acid Media," Elsevier Science BV (2003).

26. P. A. Akah and C. L. Okafor, "Blood sugar lowering effect of Vernonia amygdalina Del. in an experimental rabbit model," Phytotherapy Research 6 (1992): 171–173.

27. J. K. Crellin, Jane Phillipott, and A. L. Tommie Bass, "Diabetes Treatment 100% Remission with Steroid extract of Vernonia amygdalina," in A Reference Guide to Medicinal Plants: Herbal Medicine Past and Present (Duke University Press, 1989), 265–267.

28. Uchenna V. Okolie et al., "The Effect of Vernonia amygdalina Leaf Extract on Post Prandial Blood Glucose Concentration of Healthy Human Subjects," African Journal of Biotechnology 7 (2008): 4591–4595.

29. Abraham A. Osinubi, "Effects of Vernonia amygdalina and Chlorpropamide on Blood Glucose," Medical Journal of Islamic World Academy of Science 163: 115–119.

30. C. F. Anowi et al., "The antimicrobial activity of the crude Extract of Vernonia amygdalina Del (Asteraceae)," 2nd Nigerian Association of Pharmacists in Academia (NAPER) National Conference (October 2010).

31. H. U. Nwanjo, "Efficacy of Aqueous Leaf Extract of Vernonia amygdalina on Plasma Lipoprotein and Oxidative Status in Diabetic Rat Models," Nigerian J. of Physiological Sc. 20, 1 (2005).

32. Abraham A. Osinubi, "Effects of Vernonia amygdalina and Chlorpropamide on Blood Glucose," Medical Journal of Islamic World Academy of Science 163: 115–119.

33. C. F. Anowi et al., "The antimicrobial activity of the crude Extract of Vernonia amygdalina Del (Asteraceae)," 2nd Nigerian Association of Pharmacists in Academia (NAPER) National Conference (October 2010).

34. A. C. Igboechi and D. C. Anuforo, "Anticoagulant activities of extracts of Eupatorium odoratum and Vernonia amygdalina," The State of Medicinal Plant Research in Nigeria (1986): 313–320.

35. S. O. Awe, O. A. Olajide, and J. M. Makinde, "Effects of Allium Sativum and Vernonia amygdalina on Thrombosis in Mice," Phytotherapy Research 12, no. 1 (1998): 57–58.

36. G. Oboh, "Nutritive value and Haemolytic property (In-Vitro) of the Leaves of Vernonia amygdalina on Human Erythrocytes," Nutr. Health 18, 2 (2006): 151–60.

37. D. C. Anuforo and A. C. Igboechi, "The effect of Vernonia amygdalina, extracts on gastric emptying time in rats," The State of Medicinal Plant Research in Nigeria (1986): 321–331.

38. Aroka A. Njan et al., "Analgesic, anti-plasmodial Activity and Toxicology of V. amygdalina," Journal of Medicinal Food 11, 3 (2008): 574–581.

39. Uchechukwu Anastasia Utoh-Nedosa et al., "Excess Body Fat Elimination (Anti-Obesity) Effects of Vernonia amygdalina Leaf Extract," American Journal of Pharmacology and Toxicology (2011).

40. Uchechukwu Utoh-Nedosa, "Anti-carcinoma, Anti-obesity, Ant diabetic and Immune Defence Effects of Vernonia amygdalina Leaf Extract and Leaf Powder, in Two Human Cancer Patients," American Journal of Immunology (2011).

41. Uchechukwu Utoh-Nedosa, "Inhibition of Skin Colour Darkening; Skin Clearing; Skin Texture and Lusture Restoration; Body Calming and Body Envigorating Effects of Vernonia amygdalina leaf extract," American Journal of Pharmacology and Toxicology (2011).

42. A. U. Ugboli et al., "Medicinal application of Vernonia amygdalina Del leaf in treatment of Schistosomiasis in Mice," Nigerian Journal of Natural Products and Medicine 4 (2000): 73–75.

43. A. Tadesse et al., "The in vitro activity of Vernonia amygdalina on Leishmania aethiopica," Ethiop Med J. 31, 3 (1993): 183–189.

44. S. O. Awe, J. M. Makinde, and O. A. Olajide, "Carthatic effect of the leaf of Vernonia amygdalina," Fitoterapia 70 (1999): 161–165.

45. Abraham A. Osinubi, "Effects of Vernonia amygdalina and Chlorpropamide on Blood Glucose," Medical Journal of Islamic World Academy of Science 163: 115–119.

46. E. B. Izevbigie, "Discovery of water-soluble anticancer agents (edotides) from a vegetable found in Benin City, Nigeria," Experimental Biology and Medicines 228, 3 (2003): 293–298.

47. S. M. Kupchan et al., "Tumour inhibitors XLVII, Vernodalin and Vernomygdin, two new cytotoxic sesquiterpene lactones from Vernonia amygdalina del," J. Org. Chem 34 (1969): 3908–3911.

48. Daniel A. Oyugi et al., "Activity Markers of the Anti-Breast Carcinomer Cell Growth Fractions of Vernonia amygdalina Extract," Experimental Biology and Medicine 234 (2009): 410–417.

49. C. F. Anowi et al., "The antimicrobial activity of the crude Extract of Vernonia amygdalina Del (Asteraceae)," 2nd Nigerian Association of Pharmacists in Academia (NAPER) National Conference (October 2010).

50. T. O. Elufioye and J. M. Agbedahusi, "Antimalarial activities of Tithonia diversifolia (Asteraceae) and Crossopteryx febrifuga (Rubiaceae) on mice in vivo," Journal of Ethnopharmacology 31, 57 (2004): 1–5.

51. Aroka A. Njan et al., "Analgesic, anti-plasmodial Activity and Toxicology of V. amygdalina," Journal of Medicinal Food 11, 3 (2008): 574–581.

CHAPTER 8

Effects of Medicinal Plants of Family *Papaveraceae*, Family *Solanaceae*, and Family *Sterculiaceae*

Family *Papaveraceae* Juss.

THE *PAPAVERACEAE* ARE an economically important family of about forty-two to forty-four genera and approximately 775 to 825 known species of flowering plants in the order Ranunculales, informally known as the poppy family.[1], [2]

Most of the plants of *Papaveraceae*, the poppy family of flowering plants (order Ranunculales), are herbaceous plants; but the family also includes some woody shrubs and a genus of small tropical trees.[3] The *Papaveraceae* family includes about fifty species of the genus *Papaver* (poppy). Other genera of the *Papaveraceae* distinguished for their ornamental species include *Corydalis*, *Dicentra*, *Meconopsis*, *Eschscholzia* (California poppy), *Hunnemannia* (Mexican tulip poppy), *Dendromecon* (tree poppy), *Stylophorum*, *Chelidonium* (celandine), *Sanguinaria* (bloodroot), *Platystemon* (creamcups), *Romneya coulteri* (Matilija poppy), *Macleaya* (plumed poppy), *Stylomecon* (wind poppy), *Bocconia*, and *Eomecon* (snow poppy). The genera *Argemone* (prickly poppy), *Glaucium* (horned poppy), and *Papaver* contain weedy species. The opium poppy (*Papaver somniferum*), grown as an ornamental plant and for its edible seeds is the source of the drugs papaverine, morphine, codeine, and other opiate drugs like heroin.

Scientific Research Study on a Plant of Family *Papaveraceae*

Aqueous and ethanol extracts of *Argemone Mexicana* (family *Papaveraceae*) used in Nigerian ethnomedicine for the treatment of various skin diseases were evaluated for antimycotic activity. Minimum inhibitory concentration and maximum fungicidal concentration were determined for both extracts on *Aspergillus flavus*, *Aspergillus niger*, *Candida albicans*, *Penicillium* spp., and *Tricophyton metagrophyte*.

Both extracts produced concentration-dependent anti-mycotic activity comparable to those of ketoconazole but the water extract produced more potent activity than the ethanol extract.[4]

A preliminary phytochemical study on these extracts showed the presence of flavonoids, cardiac glycosides, saponins, tannins, and carbohydrates.[5]

Family *Solanaceae*

The family *Solanaceae* is the potato, nightshade, and "garden egg" family,[6], [7], [8] which includes some ninety-eight to one hundred genera and nearly 2,500 to 2,700 species[9], [10] in tropical and temperate regions of the world.

The *Solanaceae* or nightshades are an economically important family of flowering plants that contain annual and perennial herbs (vines, lianas, epiphytes, shrubs, and trees) planted for their food and medicinal values. Examples of plants of family *Solanaceae* are tomatoes; potato species like *Ipomea digitate* and Irish potatoes; eggplants; bell and chili peppers like *Capiscum annum* species, and tobacco.

Many members of the family contain potent alkaloids[11] like atropine, hyoscine, tomatine, solasodine, solasonine, etc., and some are highly toxic.

The *Solanaceae* consists of about ninety-eight genera and some 2,700 species with a great diversity of habitats, morphology, and ecology.

Scientific Research Studies on Plants of Family *Solanaceae*

Essential oils obtained from steam-distillation of fresh ripe Nsukka yellow pepper, *Capsicum annum* (*Solanaceae*) was separated into phenolic, acidic, and neutral fractions, which occurred in the ratio of 1:6:14. Capric acid was the single most abundant component of the essential oil.[12]

Leaf and fruit extracts of *Solanum scabrum* subsp. *Nigericum*, on analysis, yielded the alkaloids solasonine and solamargine. The extracts on hydrolysis yielded tigogenin, diosgenin, solanidine, solasodine, and sitosterol.[13]

Two cultivars of *Solanum scabrum* collected in Nigeria from highland and low land sites differed in morphological features of leaf size, orientation and pedicles, and coloration of parts of the plant. The concentration of anthocyanins in parts of the plant varied in the two cultivars but the coumarins detected in the plant appear to be the same in both cultivars.[14]

Analysis of the constituents of *Solanum dasyphylum* fruit resulted in the isolation of scopoletin (a compound known to have anticonvulsant properties) and fourteen other natural compounds.[15]

The effect of *Solanum erianthum* aqueous leaf extract on *Plasmodium berghei* was investigated in mice to assess its antimalarial property.

Results of the study showed that the extract produced a dose-dependent schizonticidal effect with chloroquine as the reference drug and a dose-related residual activity with pyrimethamine as the reference drug but did not strongly suppress established infection.[16]

The larvae of the black fly (*Simulium* spp.) (which is a vector of onchocerciasis) collected on polythene strips were dipped into extracts of *Azadirachta indica*, *Canavalia ensiformis*, and *Cestrum noctornum* for five minutes and returned to the flowing river. Control larvae were dipped in water and discharged similarly.

The number of larvae surviving on the substrate when it was recovered after two hours post-treatment was recorded for each plant extract.

Results indicated that extracts of *Azadirachta indica* were more toxic to the larvae with an LD_{50} of 1.2 mg/mL for the seed extract and 1.02 mg/mL for the leaf extract. The extract of the leaves of *Cestrum noctornum* was also toxic to the larvae with an LD_{50} of 0.58mg/mL. Secondary metabolites of the extracts indicated by phytochemical screening included tannins, phlobatannins, saponins, anthraquinones, alkaloids, and glycosides.[17]

The effect of *Datura metel* root extract (which is known to contain scopolamine, a tropane alkaloid) was evaluated on rat intestinal cholinesterase.

The root extract of *Datura metel* inhibited rat intestinal cholinesterase in vitro. This inhibition could not be reversed with concentrations of the cholinesterase substrate ruling out competitive inhibition. On the other hand, the same root extract activated cholinesterase enzyme activity at optimum higher enzyme-substrate concentrations. The presence of the leaf extract (which also produced an inhibitory response alone) potentiated the activation of cholinesterase enzyme activity at higher concentrations of the substrate by the root extract.[18] These results suggest that extracts of root and leaf extract of *Datura metel* produced a biphasic response on rat intestinal cholinesterase, inhibiting its cholinesterase enzyme activity in low concentrations (root extract or leaf extract alone) and potentiating its cholinesterase enzyme activity in high concentrations (root extract plus leaf extract). The activity of root and leaf extract of *Datura metel* also suggest that they acted by producing this biphasic response (inhibition of rat intestinal smooth muscles at low concentrations of the active constituent from the root extract alone or leaf extract alone) and cholinesterase activity activation or excitation response mediated at rat intestinal smooth muscles by the combined concentration of the active constituent from the root and leaf extract; by a mechanism which is neither adrenergic nor cholinergic.

Pulverized dry fruits of *Piper guineense* (Piperaceae), *Cyperus rotundus* (Cyperaceae), *Dennetia tripetalla* (*Annonaceae*), and *Capsicun frutescens* (*Solanaceae*) were evaluated for their protectant activity on fish against the smoked dry fish beetle, *Dennestes maculatus*. The number of live larvae, the number of live pupae and the number of live adult beetles, and dry weight loss of the fish were used as indices of activity of the powdered plant materials.

Pulverized *Dennetia tripetala* and *Piper guineense* produced the greatest protectant activity on the smoked fish.[19]

Evaluation of the antibacterial activity of essential oils from the fruits of four selected varieties of *Capsicum annum*, U-SRCP, U-RSP, U-LP, and N-YAP showed that all the essential oils exhibited antibacterial activity with N-YAP and U-SRCP exhibiting the highest activities.[20]

A study compared phytochemical and antimicrobial properties of methanol extracts of *Solanum macrocarpum* and *Solanum torvum* leaves.

The results of the study showed that *Solanum macrocarpum* and *Solanum torvum* leaf extracts contained alkaloids, steroids, and tannins; and these were present in higher concentrations in *Solanum torvum*. Extracts of both *Solanum macrocarpum* and *Solanum torvum* leaves demonstrated concentration-dependent antimicrobial properties with *Solanum torvum* extracts exhibiting slightly higher antimicrobial activities.[21]

The ability of essential oil of *Cendrus deodora* to control the fungal deterioration of two varieties of *Capsicum annum* during storage was investigated by in vitro evaluation of the effects of the oil on the molds of the two *Capsicum annum* (*Solanaceae*) varieties.

The essential oil of *Cendrus deodora* exerted strong antifungal action on the molds.[22]

The alkaloid content of the leaves of three Nigerian *Datura* species—*Datura innoxia* Mill, *Datura metel* L, and *Datura stramonium* L—was determined by TLC analysis of extracts of the leaves of these plants.

The results of the analyses showed the presence of hyoscyamine and hyoscine in the extracts as well as the presence of tropine, tigloidine, and meteloidine. An unknown alkaloid was also detected in *Datura stramonium* extract. Total alkaloid contents of the extracts were 1.75 in *Datura innoxia*, 1.22% in *Datura metel*, and 1.29% in *Datura* stramonium.[23] Given that the official drug (leaves) should contain 0.2%–0.5% of total alkaloid to be considered a standard drug, the total alkaloid content of these Nigerian *Datura* species—*Datura innoxia*, *Datura metel*, and *Datura stramonium*—qualify to be standard drugs.[24]

A comparative study evaluated the antibacterial activities of the fresh and dried fruit of *Capsicum* species (*Capsicum annum* and *Capsicum longum*) against *Staphylococus aureus*, *Salmonella typhi*, and *Bacillus subtilis* using filter disk and agar plate diffusion assay methods.

The results showed that fresh *Capsicum annum* and *Capsicum longum* potently inhibited the growth of *Staphylococus aureus* and *Salmonella typhi*, especially in the filter disc method, showing more activity than extracts of their dried counterparts. The extracts of *Capsicum frutescens* and *Capsicum grossum* (whether fresh or dry) showed no activity against any of the tested organisms.[25]

The effects of 10 g bolus consumption of *Solanum melongena* (garden egg) on some visual functions of visually active male Igbo (of Nigeria) volunteers were studied to determine the ocular effects of the active constituents of the plant.

Results showed that the pupil size was reduced by 23%, NPC was decreased by 9%, the AA was increased by 22%, the intraocular pressure dropped by 25%, and there was no effect on the VA and the habitual phoria. The miotic effect lowered the intraocular pressure and reduced the NPC which was still within the normal range. The positive correlation between the increased AA and convergence excess was concluded to provide an efficient visual mechanism, thereby suggesting that *Solanum melongena* could be of benefit to those suffering from raised intraocular pressure.[26]

A study found that glycoalkaloids, solanine possessed positive cardiotonic effects.[27] These compounds also have fungistatic effects. Ethanol extract of ripe fruit of *Solanum* spp. caused an initial transient excitatory effect followed by depression in mice. The extract also showed moderate anticonvulsive effect against leptazol-induced seisures[28] while its crushed fresh leaves had hemostatic effect in albino mice, probably mediated by its coumarin constituents.[29] The opposing or dual effects of extracts of *Solanum* species suggest biphasic effects due to initial stimulation and later inhibition at the same receptors involved in the responses.

Family *Sterculiaceae*

The *Sterculiaceae* are trees, shrubs, or herbs comprising about sixty-five genera and one thousand species that are further characterized by the presence of stellate hairs.[30]

Sterculiaceae was a family of flowering plants: based on the genus *Sterculia*. *Sterculia* genera are now placed in the family Malvaceae in the subfamilies Byttnerioideae, Dombeyoideae, Helicteroideae, and Sterculioideae.[31]

Malvaceae, the hibiscus or mallow family (order Malvales), contains some 243 genera and at least 4,225 species of herbs, shrubs, and trees.[32] Representatives occur in all except the coldest parts of the world but are most numerous in the tropics. Several species are economically important—for example, okra, *Hibiscus sabdariffa*, etc.

Examples of plants of family *Sterculiaceae* include cocoa trees and kola trees. Examples of kola trees are *Kola acuminala*, *Cola nitida*, and *Garcinia kola* tree. *Theobroma cacao* L. (family *Sterculiaceae*) is native to tropical South and Central America.[33]

Scientific Research Studies on Plants of Family *Sterculiaceae*

The antihepatotoxic activity of bioflavonoids of *Garcinia kola* seed was evaluated using four experimental poisons, carbon tetrachloride, galactosamine, amanitin, and phalloidin.

Kolaviron, a fraction of the de-fatted ethanol extract of *Garcinia kola* (family Strculiaceae) seed and two biflavones of Garcinia kola seed, GBI and GB2, potently modified the hepatotoxic effects of these poisons. The test substances (100 mg/kg) reduced thiopental-induced sleep in CCl_4-poisoned rats and greatly protected the microsomal enzyme levels in the serum of mice poisoned with phalloidin thereby suggesting that Garcinia kola seed extract has liver-protective properties.[34]

Kolaviron, a mixture of bioflavonoids of *Garcinia kola* seed extract at an intraperitoneal dose of 100 mg/kg reduced thiopental-induced sleep in the acute and chronic test models and thus protected rats against thio-acetamide-induced hepatotoxicity.[35]

Protective effects of *Garcinia kola* against paracetamol-induced hepatotoxicity were investigated in rats.

The rats received a pretreatment dose of 100 mg/kg *Garcinia kola* seed extract three times a day for five consecutive days before the administration of high doses of 800 mg/kg, 1,000 mg/kg, and 1,200 mg/kg paracetamol. The pretreatment dose of 100 mg/kg *Garcinia kola* seed extract reduced paracetamol 800 mg/kg, 1,000 mg/kg, and 1,200 mg/kg-induced lethality from 50%, 90%, and 100% to 0%, 20%, and 40% respectively.[36] The paracetamol-induced lethalities were associated with a significant reduction of liver enzymes SGOT and SGPT and histology scores.[37]

An intraperitoneal dose of 100 mg/kg of kolaviron, a mixture of C-3/C-8 linked bioflavonoids obtained from *Garcinia kola* seed extract, administered to normal and alloxan diabetic rabbits lowered the blood sugar level of the alloxan diabetic rats from 506 mg per 100 ml to 285 mg per 100 ml in twelve hours with tolbutamide acting as the positive control. It also reduced the fasting blood sugar in normoglycaemic rabbits from 115 mg per 100 ml to 65 mg per 100 ml in four hours.

Kolaviron also inhibited rat lens aldose reductase activity with an IC_{50} value of 5.4×10^{-6}. These results demonstrated antidiabetic activity of kolaviron and, by extension, antidiabetic activity of *Garcinia kola* seed extract.[38]

Three seeds used in Nigeria as hospitality snacks (given to visitors and friends as a sign of friendship or hospitality and as such could be eaten many times in a day)—*Cola acuminata*, *Cola nitida*, and *Garcinia kola*—were analyzed for their content of primary and secondary amines and their relative methylating potential due to nitosamide formation. Primary and secondary amines were determined as benzene sulphonamides by gas chromatography and thermal energy analysis (GC/TEA).

Dimethylamine, methylamine, ethylamine, and isopentylamine were detected in all kola nut varieties; and pyrrolidine, piperidine, and isobutylamine were detected in some varieties.

Methylating activity of the nitrosated kola nuts, expressed as N-nitroso-N-methylurea equivalents determined by GC/TEA, showed that methylating activity was significantly higher in kola nuts (170-490 µg/kg) than has ever been reported for a fresh plant product, suggesting the possible role of kola nut chewing in cancer etiology in countries where kola nuts are widely consumed as stimulants.[39]

The estimated average total daily intake of aliphatic amines by a typical kola nut chewer varied from 2430 µg per day to 9710 µg per day.[40]

The effect of inset pest infestation on the caffeine content of *Cola nitida* and *Cola acuminate* was investigated by comparing the caffeine content of insect-infested and uninfested nuts *Cola nitida* and *Cola acuminata* collected from four geographical zones of Nigeria using high-performance liquid chromatography (HPLC).

The results showed that insect infestation had no significant effect on the caffeine content of kola nut samples analyzed.[41]

Capillary electrophoresis determination of biflavanones GB1, GB2, GB1-glycoside, and kolaflavanone in 'tea' (water extract) and two alcohol beverage formulations of *Garcinia kola* (with optimum separation conditions of 100 mM borate, pH 9.5 running buffer, which gave baseline resolution of all four components in twelve minutes) showed that the fingerprint of the biflavanones (linear calibration ranges for each component was between 2.5 µg/mL and 1,000 µg/mL and limits of detection between 3 and 6 µg/mL) in the aqueous "tea" and two ethanol "beverage" formulations were similar. The concentrations of the four biflavanones were up to 50% higher in the ethanol formulations than in the aqueous formulation and the major biflavanone in all three formulations was GB128.

Waltheria indica (family *Sterculiaceae*) used in Nigerian traditional medicine for the treatment of gonorrhea, skin diseases, internal hemorrhage, pain relief, infertility, and diarrhea was studied to determine the macroscopic, microscopic chemomicroscopic data on anatomical sections of the plant. Preliminary phytochemical screening of extract of the powdered leaves of the plant was also done to find out its phytochemical constituents.

Microscopic studies showed the presence of calcium oxalate crystals, anisocytic stomata, and groups of unicellular stellate covering trichomes. Phytochemical screening showed the presence of saponins, alkaloids, steroids, tannins, flavonoids, terpenes, sugars, and mucillages.[42]

The traditional use parts of *Waltheria indica* for wound healing prompted screening of the aqueous and ethanol extracts of the leaves of *Waltheria indica* for antimicrobial activity against the bacteria *Bacillus cereus* (ATCC 14579), *Escherichia coli* (NCTC10418), *Staphylococus aureus* (ATCC17079), and clinical isolates of *Pseudomonas aeruginosa* and *Salmonella typhi* and two fungi, *Candida albicans* and *Aspergillus niger*, using the paper disc diffusion method.

The results showed that both the water and the ethanol extracts of *Waltheria indica* inhibited each of the bacterial organisms to some degree and the ethanol extract showed more potent antibacterial activity than the aqueous extract of *Waltheria indica*. Both the ethanol extract and aqueous extracts of *Waltheria indica* showed the least antibacterial activity on *Escherichia coli* and *Salmonella typhi*.[43]

Central inhibitory activity of the aqueous extract of *Crinum gigantum* was exhibited in experimental rats and mice. The intraperitoneal and oral LD_{50} of *Crinum gigantum* in mice were 627 and 1,468. When given by the intraperitoneal route at doses of 6.25 mg/kg, 12.5 mg/kg, and 25 mg/kg to rats, the aqueous extract of *Crinum gigantum* prolonged pentobarbital sleeping time and in mice, reduced spontaneous motor activity; decreased exploratory activity, and reduced amphetamine-induced stereotype behavior. These results suggested that some active principles of extracts of *Crinum gigantum* possess some sedative activity.[44]

Five percent aqueous and methanol leaf and stem bark extracts of *Garcinia kola* exhibited anti-fungal activities on purulent fungal organisms from human ocular discharges in Lagos University Teaching Hospital.[45]

Extracts and fractions of *Garcinia kola* have been shown in different studies to produce predominantly inhibitory effects, some of which are (a) antispasmodic effects[20]; (b) inhibition of drug metabolism;[46] antibacterial, antifungal, and antimicrobial[47, 48, 49, 50] properties; (d) cough-depressant effects;[51] (e) inhibition of gastric acid secretion beyond basal levels;[52, 53, 54] (f) production of powerful anti-oxidant properties;[55] and (g) production of powerful liver-protective effects against liver damage by poisons like aminofluerene,[56] D-galactosamine,[57] or genotoxicity or DNA damage by oxidative stress.[58, 59] Different organic solvents produced varying degrees of the same results of the effects of Garcinia cola extracts[60, 61] and some solvents like methanol produced effects that are opposite[62] to the effect of the water extract of *Garcinia kola* seed, a seed actually eaten frequently by its native users in Nigeria for its medicinal properties.

Organic solvents used to dissolve extracts of other plants behave similarly. For example, both the water and the ethanol extracts of *Waltheria indica* inhibited each of the bacterial organisms used to evaluate the antibacterial activity of *Waltheria indica* to some degree, but the ethanol extract showed more potent antibacterial activity than the aqueous extract of *Waltheria indica*.[63]

Effect of atropine or ranitidine on the action of aqueous *Garcinia kola* seed extract on gastric acid secretion in rats indicated the site of action of *Garcinia kola* extracts. Water extract of *Garcinia kola* seed dose-dependently inhibited increases in gastric acid secretion beyond normal levels. The inhibition of gastric acid secretion by atropine and ranitidine each increased with increasing doses of aqueous *Garcinia kola* extract which demonstrated a synergistic inhibition of gastric acid secretion by aqueous *Garcinia kola* extract and atropine or ranitidine.

Thus, aqueous *Garcinia kola* seed extract inhibited increases in gastric acid secretion beyond basal levels on its own and produced a dose-dependent marked synergistic inhibition of gastric acid secretion with atropine (a muscarinic antagonist) and ranitidine (a histamine (H2)-receptor antagonist, also regarded as a serotonin receptor antagonist). Partial inhibition of gastric acid secretion by atropine or ranitidine ruled out excitatory cholinergic muscarinic and histamine (H2)-receptor activity as mediators of gastric acid secretion and suggested serotonin receptors as the site of inhibition of gastric acid secretion by atropine, ranitidine, and aqueous *Garcinia kola* seed extract. Atropine was more efficacious than ranitidine in inhibition of gastric acid secretion in the test rats (reducing the acidity of the gastric effluent produced under the effect of 2 mg/mL aqueous *Garcinia kola* seed extract from 1.5 mM to 1 mM (while ranitidine reduced it from 1.5 mM to 1.45 mM). These results suggest that serotonin receptor was the site of inhibition of gastric acid secretion by atropine, ranitidine, and aqueous *Garcinia kola* seed extract.

A study that estimated the secondary metabolites in *Garcinia kola* seed noted that *Garcinia kola* seed extract showed the presence of tannin (0.69 ± 0.01), saponin (15.79 ± 0.28), oxalate (1.707 ± 0.13), cryogenic glycosides (59.56 ± 0.05), and cardiac glycosides (67.10 ± 0.03 mg per 100 g dry matter).[64]

References

1. Wikipedia, "Papaveraceae," https://en.wikipedia.org/wiki/Papaveraceae.
2. Britannica, "Papaveraceae, Description, Characteristics and Examples," accessed September 21, 2018, https://www.britannica.com/plant/Papaveraceae.
3. C. F. Anowi, I. M. Ononiwu, and U. A. Utoh-Nedosa, "Effect of Atropine or Ranitidine on the action of Aqueous Garcinia kola Seed Extract, on Gastric Acid Secretion in Rats," International Journal of Advances in Pharmacy, Biology and Chemistry 3, 1 (2014): 180–183.
4. A. Agunu et al., "Antimycotic activity of Argemone Mexicana," Nigerian Journal of Natural Products and Medicine 7 (2003): 72.
5. Ibid.
6. Britannica, "Solanaceae/Plant family, accessed September 21, 2018, www.britannica.com/plant/Solanaceae.
7. Wikipedia, "Solanaceae," accessed September 21, 2018, https://en.wikipedia.org/wiki/Solanaceae.
8. Thomas J. Elpel's Web World Portal, "Nightshade Family. Identify plants, flowers," Wildflowers-and-Weeds.com, accessed September 21, 2018, https://www.wildflowers-and-weeds.com/Plant_Families/Solanaceae.htm.
9. Britannica, "Solanaceae/Plant family, accessed September 21, 2018, www.britannica.com/plant/Solanaceae.
10. Wikipedia, "Solanaceae," accessed September 21, 2018, https://en.wikipedia.org/wiki/Solanaceae.
11. Ibid.
12. E. O. P. Agbakwuru et al., "The fragrant principles of the Nsukka yellow pepper, Capsicum annum (Solanaceae): Studies on the essential oil and its acidic fractions," Research into Medicinal Plants Newsletter 27, 8 and 9 (1983): 65.
13. H. Nuhu and A. Ghani, "Alkaloid content of the leaves of three Nigerian Datura species," Nigerian Journal of Natural Products and Medicine 6 (2002): 15.
14. Z. O. Gbile and S. K. Adesina, "Taxonomy and Chemistry of Nigerian Solanum scabrum," Fitoterapia 56, 1 (1985): 11–16.
15. S. K. Adesina, "Constituents of Solanum dasyphylum fruit," Journal of Natural Products 49, 1 (1985): 147.
16. J. M, Makinde, P. O. Obih, and A. A. Jimoh, "Effect of Solanum erianthum aqueous leaf extract on Plasmodium berghei in mice," African Journal of Medicine and Medical Sciences 16 (1987): 193–196.
17. J. A. Onah, D. Kumsah, and J. O. Abah, "Evaluation on the plant extracts (Azadirachta indica, Canavalia ensiformis and Cestrum noctornum) on immature states and vectors of Onchocerciasis (Simuiium spp.)," 8th International Symposium on Medicinal Plants (1992): 89.
18. E. Prabhakar and N. V. Nanda Kumar, "Potentiating action of Datura metel Linn. root extract on rat intestinal cholinesterase," Phytotherapy Research 6 (1992): 160–162.
19. C. O. Aderire and L. Lajide, "Effect of pulverised plant materials on fish damage and growth performance of the fish beetle, Dennestes maculatus," Essential Occasional Publication 31 (1998): 215–218.

20. C. S. Odoemena, K. E. Akpabio, and C. P. Nneji, Antibacterial Activity of Essential oils from four selected varieties of Capsicum annum," Nigerian Journal of Natural Products and Medicine 2 (1998): 49–51.

21. E. O. Ajaiyeoba, "Comparative phytochemical and antimicrobial studies of Solanum macrocarpum and Solanum torvum leaves," Fitotherapia 70 (1999): 184–186.

22. E. P. Essien and J. P. Essien, "Control of fungal deterioration of two varieties of Capssicum annum during storage by the essential oil of Cendrus deodora," Nigerian Journal of Natural Products and Medicine 4 (2000): 62–64.

23. H. Nuhu and A. Ghani, "Alkaloid content of the leaves of three Nigerian Datura species," Nigerian Journal of Natural Products and Medicine 6 (2002): 15.

24. Ibid.

25. S. Umukoro and R. B. Ashorobi, "Comparative study of antibacterial activities of the fresh and dried fruit of Capsicum species," Nigerian Journal of Health and Biomedical Sciences 2, 2 (2003): 90–93.

26. S. A. Igwe, D. N. Akunyili, and C. Ogbogu, "Effects of Solanum melongena (garden egg) on some visual functions of visually active Igbos of Nigeria," Journal of Ethnopharmacology 86, 2–3 (2003): 135–138.

27. W. W. A. Bergers and G. M. Alink, "Toxic effects of glycoalkaloids Solanine and Tomatine on cultured neonatal rats," Toxicol. Letters 6 (1980): 29–32.

28. S. K. Adesina, "Constituents of Solanum dasyphylum fruit," Journal of Natural Products 49, 1 (1985): 147.

29. Z. O. Gbile and S. K. Adesina, "Taxonomy and Chemistry of Nigerian Solanum scabrum," Fitoterapia 56, 1 (1985): 11–16.

30. "Sterculiaceae," University of Hawaii, accessed September 21, 2018, www.botany.hawaii.edu/faculty/carr/sterculi.htm.

31. Wikipedia, "Sterculiaceae," accessed September 21, 2018, https://en.wikipedia.org/wiki/Sterculiaceae.

32. Britannica, "Malvaceae/plant family," accesses September 21, 2018, https://www.britannica.com/plant/Malvaceae.

33. K. P. Prabhakaran Nair, "Sterculiaceae: Cocoa (Teobbroma L)," in The Agronomy and Economy of Important Tree Crops of the Developing World, accessed September 21, 2018, https://www.sciencedirect.com/.../sterculiaceae.

34. M. M. Iwu et al., "Evaluation of the anti-hepatotoxic activity of bioflavonoids of Garcinia kola seed," Journal of Ethnopharmacology 21, 2 (1987): 127–138.

35. M. M. Iwu et al., "Prevention of Thioacetamide-induced hepatotoxicity by bioflavonoids of Garcinia kola seed," Phytotherapy Research 4, 4 (1990): 157–159.

36. A. Akintonwa and A. R. Essien "Protective effects of Garcinia kola against paracetamol-induced hepatotoxicity," Journal of Ethnopharmacology 29, 2 (1990): 207–211.

37. Ibid.

38. M. M. Iwu et al., "Antidiabetic and Aldose Reductase Activities of Biflavonones of Garcinia cola," Journal of Pharmacology 42, 4 (1990): 290–292.

39. S. E. Atawodi et al., "Nitrostable amines and nitrosamide formation in natural stimulants Cola acuminata, Cola nitida and Garcinia kola," Food Chemistry and Toxicology 33, 8 (1995): 625–630.

40. Ibid.

41. V. O. Makanju and H. Maskill, "Effect of inset pest infestation on the caffeine content of Cola nitida and Cola acuminata," Nigerian Journal of Natural Products and Medicine 1, 1 (1997): 25–28.

42. U. A. Katsayal, Z. Mohammed, and M. Shok, "Pharmacognostic Studies on the leaves of Waltheria indica," Nigerian Journal of Botany 15 (2002): 47–52.

43. U. A. Katsayal et al., "Preliminary phytochemical screening of the leaves of Waltheria indica," Journal of Pharmaceutical and Allied Sciences 1 (2003): 80–84.

44. S. Amos et al., "Central inhibitory activity of the aqueous extract of Crinum gigantum," Fitotherapia 74, 1–2 (2003): 23–28.

45. F. Obuekwe and N. D. Onwukaeme, "Anti-fungal activities of Garcinia kola Extracts on purulent human ocular discharges in Lagos University Teaching Hospital, Lagos Herkel," Nigerian Quarterly Journal of Hospital Medicine 14, 1 (2004): 112–114.

46. V. B. Braide, "Inhibition of drug metabolism by flavonoid extract (Kolaviron) of Garcinia kola seeds in the rat," Phytotherapy Research 1 (1991).

47. F. Obuekwe and N. D. Onwukaeme, "Phytochemical analysis and anti-microbial activities of the leaf and stem bark of extracts of Garcinia kola Herkel (Family Guttiferae)," Pakistan Journal of Science Research 47, 2 (2004): 160–162.

48. Uzondu Akueyinwa, Uchechukwu A. Utoh-Nedosa, and Chinedu Fred Anowi, "Comparison of the antimicrobial activities of n-hexane and diethyl ether extracts of Garcinia kola Heckel (bitter kola) seed," IJAPBC (Int. J. of Advances in Pharmacy, Biology and Chemistry) 3, 1 (January–March 2014).

49. Uzondu Akueyinwa et al., "Phytochemical screening and antimicrobial evaluation of diethyl ether extract of Garcinia kola; Heckel (bitter kola) seed," IJRPC (International Journal of Research in Pharmacy and Chemistry) 4, 2 (2014): 237–242.

50. L. E. Uzondu Akueyinwa, U. A. Utoh-Nedosa, and Chinedu Fredrick Anowi, "Phytochemical screening and antimicrobial evaluation of n-hexane extract of Garcinia kola Heckel (bitter kola) seed," International Journal of Pharmacy 4, 4 (2014).

51. U. A. Utoh-Nedosa et al., "Cough Suppressant, Cough Expectorant and Irritant Throat-clearing Properties of Garcinia cola seed extract, Inventi Rapid: Planta Activa, no. 1 (2011).

52. C. F. Anowi, I. M. Ononiwu, and U. A. Utoh-Nedosa, "Comparison of the Effect of Methylene Chloride Extract and Aqueous Extract of Garcinia kola (Heckel) Seed on Gastric Acid Secretion in Rats," IJRPC (International Journal of Research in Pharmacy and Chemistry) 3, 3 (2013): 530–532.

53. Chinedu F. Anowi et al., "Comparative profile of the effects of four extracts of Garcinia cola seed on gastric acid secretion in rats," Pharmanest, an international Journal of Advances in Pharmaceutical Sciences 4, 5 (2013): 1021–1028.

54. C. F. Anowi, I. M. Ononiwu, and U. A. Utoh-Nedosa, "Effect of Atropine or Ranitidine on the action of Aqueous Garcinia kola Seed Extract, on Gastric Acid Secretion in Rats," International Journal of Advances in Pharmacy, Biology and Chemistry 3, 1 (2014): 180–183.

55. K. Tarashma, Akaya Takaya, and M. Niwa, "Powerful antioxidant agents based on Garcinic acid from Garcinia kola, Bio-organism and Medicinal Chemistry 10, 5 (2002): 1619–1625.

56. O. A. Odunola et al., "Protection Against 2-acetyl aminofluerene-induced toxicity in mice by garlic (Allium sativum), bitter kola (Garcinia kola) and Honey," African Journal of Medical Science 34, 2 (2005): 167–172.

57. O. A. Adaramoye and E. O. Adeyemi, "Hepatoprotection of D-galactosamine-induced toxicity in mice by purified fractions from Garcinia kola seeds," Basal Clinical Pharmacology and Toxicology 98, 2 (2006): 132–141.

58. E. O. Farombi, P. Moller, and L. O. Dragsted, "Ex-vivo and In-vitro Protective Effects of Kolaviron against Oxygen-Derived Radical-Induced DNA Damage in Human Lymphocytes and Rat Liver cells," Cell Biology and Toxicology 20, 2 (2004): 71–82.

59. E. O. Farombi et al., "Chemoprevention of Aflatoxin B1-induced genotoxicity and Hepatic Oxidative Damage in Rats by Kolaviron, a Natural Bi-flavonoid of Garcinia kola Seeds," European Journal of Cancer Prevention 14, 3 (2005): 207–214.

60. Chinedi F. Anowi et al., "Effect of gastric acid secretion in rats of combining methanol with methylene chloride (50/50) as solvent for Garcinia kola seed extract," Int. Res. J. Pharmacy and Pharmacology 3, 3 (2013).

61. Uzondu Akueyinwa, Uchechukwu A. Utoh-Nedosa, and Chinedu Fred Anowi, "Comparison of the antimicrobial activities of n-hexane and diethyl ether extracts of Garcinia kola Heckel (bitter kola) seed," IJAPBC (Int. J. of Advances in Pharmacy, Biology and Chemistry) 3, 1 (January–March 2014).

62. Chinedu F. Anowi et al., "Comparative profile of the effects of four extracts of Garcinia cola seed on gastric acid secretion in rats," Pharmanest, an international Journal of Advances in Pharmaceutical Sciences 4, 5 (2013): 1021–1028.

63. U. A. Katsayal et al., "Preliminary phytochemical screening of the leaves of Waltheria indica," Journal of Pharmaceutical and Allied Sciences 1 (2003): 80–84.

64. C. C. Monago and V. Akhidue, "Estimation of Tannin, Saponin, Oxalate, Cyagenic Glycosides and Cardiac Glycosides in Garcinia kola," Journal of Applied Sciences and Environmental Management 6, 1 (2002): 22–25.

CHAPTER 9

Effects of Extracts and Juices of Plants of Family *Apocynaceae*

Family *Apocynaceae*

P LANTS OF FAMILY *Apocynaceae* are herbs, shrubs, and trees that resemble *Rauwolfia* species. They usually produce a white latex or milky sap[1] when injured or incised. Plants of family *Apocynaceae* belong to the dogbane family of flowering plants of the gentian order (Gentianales), including more than 411 to 415 genera[2], [3] and about 1,500 to 4,600 species of trees, shrubs, woody vines, and herbs distributed primarily in tropical and subtropical areas of the world.[4] The *Apocynaceae* are also plants of the periwinkle family,[5] which is a large family that includes many of the most well-known tropical ornamental plants like rose periwinkle, milkweed, oleander,[6] frangipani, *Allamanda*, *Mandevilla*, and *Rauwolfia vomitura*. Reserpine is an important rauwolfian alkaloid from a member of this family. Many genera of the *Apocynaceae* family produce cardiac glycosides that are useful medically.[7]

Scientific Researches on Plants of Family *Apocynaceae*

Preliminary biological and phytochemical investigation of ten extracts of two Nigerian medicinal plants, *Pleioceras barteri* Baill (Apocynaceae) and *Marsdenia latifolia* Schum (Asclepidiaceae), showed that nine of the extracts gave positive tests for alkaloids, four for flavonoids, five for saponins, two for tannins, and four for steroids. *Pleioceras barteri* showed abortifacient property while extracts of both plants showed antibacterial activity.[8]

The roots of *Rauwolfia volkensii* yielded twenty-six alkaloids that belonged to five main groups made up of sarpagan; akuammicine, and heteroyohimbine with derived oxindole; anhydronium bases; yohimbine with 18-hydroxy-yohimbine and its derived esters; and dihyroindole alkaloids.

The principal alkaloids identified were ajmaline (0.08%) and reserpiline (0.15%). The reserpine yield was very low (0.0007%).[9]

Chromogenic reactions of forty-one rauwolfian alkaloids after separation by thin-layer chromatography identified dihydroindole alkaloids as the most definable group. Aricine; 10, 11-dimethoxyheteroyohimbines; sapagine ar-substituted 18-hydroxy-yohimbines; and their esters were distinguishable using various reagents.[10]

Autonomic pharmacology of echitamine, an alkaloid from *Alstonia boonei* (family *Apocynaceae*) was investigated in rats, rabbits, guinea pigs, and cats. The results of the study showed that the alkaloid echitamine depressed or abolished the amplitude of spontaneous myogenic contractions of rat isolated portal vein; the rabbit isolated duodenum and the electrically stimulated or nor-adrenaline-induced constriction of the rabbit isolated perfused central ear artery, in a concentration-dependent manner.

Echitamine also inhibited or abolished agonist-induced (acetylcholine, histamine, serotonin, nicotine, K^+, or Ba^{2+}) contractions of guinea pig ileum; electrically stimulated contractions of chick isolated oesophagus; and guinea pig-isolated vas deferens in a dose-dependent manner. Echitamine also dose-dependently depressed or abolished relaxations of the rabbit isolated duodenum; depressed systemic arterial blood pressure of normotensive cats and blocked neuromuscular transmission in the various muscle-nerve transmissions.

The depressor (hypotensive) effect of echitamine in the anesthetized cat was not modified by cervical bilateral vagotomy, atropinisation, or mepyramine treatment. The hypotensive effect of echitamine was suggested not to have been mediated via cholinergic mechanisms or histamine H_1 receptor stimulation.[11]

Aqueous extract of the stem bark of *Alsonia boonei* (*Apocynaceae*) exhibited contractile activity on isolated rat stomach strip and guinea pig ileum.[12] This effect was more pronounced on rat stomach strip than guinea pig ileum.[13]

The stem bark extract of *Alstonia boonei* also showed anticomplement activity on the human complement system and polymorphonuclear leucocytes.[14] *Alstonia boonei* stem bark extract also demonstrated anti-inflammatory, antipyretic, and analgesic properties.

The *Alstonia boonei* stem bark extract inhibited carrageenan-induced paw edema, cotton pellet granuloma, and acetic acid-induced vascular edema.[7] The alcoholic root extract of *Alstonia boonei* inhibited egg white-induced rat paw edema.[15]

Extracts of *Alstonia boonei* also showed potential anti-helminthic activity by their inhibition of glutathione-s-transferases (GSTs) from parasitic nematodes.[16]

Boiling water extracts of *Picrallima nitida* bark showed trypanosomacidal action comparable to that of diminazene acturate in the treatment of experimental trypanosomiasis.[17]

Amides were isolated from extracts of the stem and root bark of *Zanthoxylum rubescens*. The amides from the stem bark were identified as rubemamide and rubemamin while the amides isolated from the root bark were identified as dioxamide and domain. Lupeol and arnottianamide were also isolated from the root extract. Both the stem and root back also yielded the known aromatic amide zanthomamide.[18]

Evaluation of the in vitro antimalarial activity of fruit, rind, and stem bark extracts of *Picralima nitida* showed that they had high inhibitory activity against drug-resistant clones of *Plasmodium falciparum* at doses of 3.2-32 µg/mL. The dichloromethane extract of the rind was the most active and had an IC_{50} value of 0.61 ug/mL for the Indochina (W-2) clone and 2.41 µg/mL for the Sierra Leone (D-6) clone of Plasmodium falciparum. An alkaloid isolated from the methanol extract of the stem bark of *Picralima nitida* gave an IC_{50} value of 2.0 mg/mL and 1.23 µg/mL for the Indochina (W-2) and Sierra Leone (D-6) clones.[19]

Crude root extract and n-hexane, chloroform, ethylacetate and n-butanol fractions of *Pleioceras barteri* root extract showed activity against nine species of bacteria and showed low antifungal activity. Of the sensitive bacteria, *B. subtilis* was the most susceptible to the extracts while *P. vulgaris* and *S. marcescens* were the least susceptible.[20]

Crude extracts of dried root of *Rauwolfia vomitoria* administered orally to ten Nigerian psychiatric inpatients at doses of up to 800 mg per day in divided doses showed antipsychotic effects. The antipsychotic effects of the extract were dose-dependent when administered three times a day and were accompanied by minimal side effects as they were without serious incidences of extrapyramidal symptoms.

Physical examination and laboratory parameters observed tended to correlate with the theory that *Rauwolfia vomitoria* accumulate in the plasma.[21]

Biochemical effects of water extracts of pink and white varieties of *Catharantus roseus*, *Calistermom citrinus*, and *Persea americana* (family *Apocynaceae*) were evaluated in rats.

Boiled distilled water extracts of 20 g of each herb in 100 mL of water were administered orally to test rats, and distilled water was administered to control rats. The levels of blood glucose, lipids, and the activities of transaminases were determined.

Extracts of each of the three plants potently increased blood cholesterol but did not affect HDL-cholesterol levels. None of the aqueous extracts of the pink variety of *Catharantus roseus*, *Calistermom citrinus*, and *Persea americana* affected the activity of transaminases, but the extract of white *Catharantus roseus* increased the aspartate transaminase activity of the rats.

Only the extract of the pink variety of *Catharantus roseus* potently decreased blood glucose levels, suggesting that of the three plants whose extracts were tested, only the extract of the pink variety of *Catharantus roseus* has hypoglycaemic activity.[22]

Anti-inflammatory and antinociceptive activities from chloroform extract of *Voacanga africana* (family *Apocynaceae*) leaf were evaluated in mice and rats. In a dose-dependent manner, the extract (50-150 mg/kg), inhibited carrageenin-induced rat paw edema and inhibited cotton granuloma and vascular permeability induced in rat duodenum by acetic acid, suggesting that the extract had anti-inflammatory properties.

The extract similarly showed good analgesic properties by inhibiting the neurologic first phase and the second phase of the formalin-induced pain; it also produced high inhibition of writhing in acetic acid-induced pain in mice and protected tested animals against pain tested by the flick, hot-plate, and limb-withdrawal tests.[23]

Sarmentocide-A isolated from the extract of the seeds of *Strophantus sarmentosus* (family *Apocynaceae*) was tested on rabbit heart preparation. It increased the force and rate of heart contraction which compared favorably with those of digoxin. The increase in the force and rate of heart contraction produced by both sarmentocide and digoxin was antagonized by potassium chloride solution.[24]

Extracts of *Picralima nitida* demonstrated hypoglycaemic properties by a mechanism independent of the availability of insulin from pancreatic β-cell.[25]

Aqueous and ethanol extracts of leaves and bark of *Alstonia boonei* were investigated for their medical values as a source of antimalarial drugs and as a source of vitamin C using infrared and ultraviolet spectrophotometers to determine compounds present in the extracts.

Confirmed components of the extracts included quinolinic compounds, vitamin C, and ethers. The pH of the extract in the water at 35°C was 5.8.[26]

An oral dose of 1.2 g/kg of aqueous extract of the leaves of *Rauwolfia vomitoria* (*Apocynacea*) produced a decrease of temperature from 42.0°C to 40°C in two hours in rabbits infected with *Klebsiella aerogenes*.[27]

Alstonine, a heteroyohimbine-type alkaloid isolated from a Nigerian botanical remedy, exhibited an antipsychotic-like profile by inhibiting amphetamine-induced lethality, apomorphine-induced stereotypy, and potentiating barbiturate-induced sleeping time.

Atypical features of alstonine observed were the prevention of haloperidol-induced catalepsy and lack of direct interaction with D1, D2, and 5-HT2A receptors classically linked to antipsychotic mechanism of action.[28]

Acaricidal efficacy of the aqueous stem bark extract of *Adenium obesum* (family *Apocynaceae*) was studied on larvae, nymph, adult males, and fully engorged females of two cattle ticks, *Boophilus* spp. and *Amblyomma* spp.

The results of the study showed concentration-dependent toxicity of the stem bark extract on larval ticks with LC_{50} of 18.62 ± 1.05 mg/mL and 27.54 ± 0.92 mg/mL for *Amblyomma* and *Boophilus* species respectively and LD_{50} of 31.62 ± 2.84 mg/mL and 51.29 ± 3.01 mg/mL for adult and nymph *Amblyomma* spp. and *Boophilus* species respectively. The proportion of extract-treated engorged female ticks that laid viable eggs was higher than that of those that did not lay any eggs ($P < 0.05$). The results suggested that the aqueous stem bark extract of *Adenium obesum* had acaricidal properties.[29]

Hot and cold aqueous and ethanol extracts of the whole root, root bark, and root wood of *Landolphia owerrience* (family *Apocynaceae*) were evaluated for antibacterial activity using agar well diffusion and macro-broth dilution methods respectively.

Ethanol and aqueous extracts of root bark of *Landolphia owerrience* were moderately active on the organisms while the wood extracts were inactive. Of the nine extracts prepared, 66.7% demonstrated antibacterial activity against *Staphylococcus aureus* ATCC 12600; and 55.6% were active to varying degrees against Pseudomonas aeruginosa ATCC 10145 and local isolates of *Pseudomonas aeruginosa*, *Escherichia coli*, and *Salmonella typhi*; 44.4% were active against *Proteus* spp.; 33.3% were active against *Bacillus subtillis*; and 22.2% were active against *Escherichia coli* ATCC 11775.

The MIC values determined for the macro-broth diluted whole-root extract samples was 0.39-50 mg/ml while that determined for the ethanol extract of the whole root used in the agar well samples was 0.78-50 mg/mL, which suggested that the agar well samples produced lower activity. The reverse occurred with the control drug gentamycin whose agar well samples had a MIC value of 0.125-8.0 g/mL, and its macro-broth diluted samples had the MIC value of 0.125-64 g/mL.

The strong antibacterial activity of the ethanol extract of the root of *Landolphia owerrience* authenticated its similar use in Nigerian traditional medicine.[30]

The basic fraction of the methanol extract of the stem bark of *Picralima nitida* (*Apocynaceae*) showed high antibacterial activity against a wide range of gram-positive bacteria and fungi but had low activity against gram-negative bacteria. Its MIC value against *Staphlococcus aureus* was similar to that of the control drug ampicillin.

Its MIC values against *Staphlococcus aureus*, *Aspergillus flavus*, and *Aspergillus niger* were lower than that of the control drug tioconazole. Values of the minimum bactericidal concentration of the basic fraction against microorganisms tested were generally higher than those of ampicillin and gentamycin. These results indicate high antimicrobial activity of the basic fraction of the methanol extract of the stem bark of *Picralima nitida*.[31]

The basic fraction of the methanol extract of stem bark of *Picralima nitida* had been shown to have potent fungicidal activity against many fungi (but not *Aspergillus flavus* and *Aspergillus niger*). The basic alkaloidal fraction of stem bark extracts of *Picralima nitida* was therefore evaluated for dermal and acute toxicity in animals.

Acute intraperitoneal toxicity tests showed a dose-dependent inflammation and necrosis of liver hepatocytes; decrease in neutrophil count and increase in lymphocyte count. However, dermal tests showed that the extract did not cause reddening, skin inflammation, sensitization, or death to the tested animals.[32]

The indole alkaloid alstonine, which is the major component of extracts of *Rauwolfia vomitoria* (*Apocynaceae*) used by Nigerian traditional medicine practitioners for the treatment of psychosis, was evaluated for proconvulsant activity by comparing its convulsant activity with those of an anti-psychotic drug, clozapine, through repetitive administration over thirty days.

The results of the study showed that unlike clozapine, alstonine did not exhibit pro-convulsant activity.[33]

The hole-board and light/dark models were used to determine if alstonine possessed anxiolytic properties in mice. The participation of dopamine D1, glutamate NMDA, serotonin 5-HT$_{2A/2C}$, and aminobutyric acid GABA receptors in the antipsychotic effects of alstonine were also evaluated.

The results of the study showed that alstonine clearly behaved like an anxiolytic in both hole-board and light/dark tests. Pre-treatment with the 5-HT$_{2A/2C}$ serotonin receptor antagonist ritanserin reversed the effects of alstonine in both the hole-board and light/dark models suggesting the involvement of serotonin 5-HT$_{2A/2}$ receptors in the mechanism of anxiolytic effects of the antipsychotic alkaloid alstonine.[34]

Other results of the study showed that alstonine partially reversed the increase in locomotion induced by MK-801 in the hole-board test and that alstonine also partially reversed the MK-801-induced hyperlocomotion in motor activity apparatus.[35]

These results suggest that MK-801 produced increased locomotion in the hole-board model and hyperlocomotion in motor activity apparatus by partially blocking β sub-units and hyper-stimulating α-subunits of 5-HT$_{2A/2C}$ serotonin receptors of the brain; the hyperstimulation of 5-HT$_{2A/2C}$ receptors of brain areas that control locomotion thereby effected hyperlocomotion of the mice.

Alstonine produced a partial reversal of the increase in locomotion induced by MK-801 in the hole-board test and also produced a partial reversal of the MK-801-induced hyperlocomotion in motor activity apparatus by inhibiting the blocking effect of MK-801 at β subunits of serotonin receptors of the brain but was unable to inhibit the hyperexcitatory effect of MK-801 on α subunits of brain 5-HT$_{2A/2C}$ serotonin receptors; thereby achieving only a partial block of the increased locomotion stimulated by Mk-801. These results also suggest that glutamate NMDA receptors are parts or whole of serotonin receptors and that total inhibition of glutamate NMDA-induced hyperactivity involves total inhibition of excitation of α-subunits of serotonin receptors of the tissue or organ in question.

References

1. UH Botany, "Flowering Plant Families," www www.botany.hawaii.edu/faculty/carr/apocyn.htm.
2. Britannica, "Apocynaceae/plant family," accessed September 27, 2018, https://www.britannica.com/plant/Apocynaceae.
3. "Apocynaceae," Eeob.iastate.ed, accessed September 27, 2018, https://www.eeob.iastate.edu/classes/bio366/families/Apocynaceae.pdf.
4. Britannica, "Apocynaceae/plant family," accessed September 27, 2018, https://www.britannica.com/plant/Apocynaceae.
5. "Apocynaceae Seed," accessed September 27, 2018, theseedsite.co.uk/apocynaceae.html.
6. "Apocynaceae," Eeob.iastate.ed, accessed September 27, 2018, https://www.eeob.iastate.edu/classes/bio366/families/Apocynaceae.pdf.
7. Ibid.
8. A. J. Aladesanmi, A. Sofowora, and J. D. Leary, "Preliminary biological and phytochemical investigation of two Nigerian medicinal plants," International Journal of Crude Drug Research 24, 3 (1985): 147–153.
9. B. A. Akinloye and W. E. Court, "The alkaloids of Rauwolfia volkensii," Journal of Ethnopharmacology 4 (1981): 99–109.
10. W. E. Court and M. M. Iwu, "Chromogenic reactions of Rauwolfian alkaloids after separation by thin-layer chromatography," Journal of Chromatography 187, 1 (1980): 199–207.
11. John A. O. Ojewale, "Autonomic pharmacology of Echitamine, an alkaloid from Alstonia boonei De Wild," Fitotherapia 54, 3 (1983): 99–113.
12. O. B. Taiwo and J. M. Makinde, "Contractile activity of Alstonia boonei stem bark extract on isolated rat stomach strip and guinea pig ileum," Indian J. of Pharmacol 28, 2 (1996): 110–2.
13. Ibid.
14. O. B. Taiwo, A. J. J. Van Den Berg, and B. H. Kores, "Activity of the stem bark extract of Alstonia boonei De Wild (Apocynaceae) on human complement and polymorphonuclear leucocytes," Indian J. Pharmacol 30, 3 (1998): 169–174.
15. P. O. Osadebe, "Anti-inflammatory properties of the root bark of Alstonia boonei," Nigerian J. of Natural Products and Medicine 6 (2002): 39–41.
16. B. B. Fakae et al., "Inhibition of glutathione-s-transferases (GSTs) from parasitic nematodes by extracts from traditional Nigerian medicinal plant," Phytother Res. 14, 8 (2000): 630–634.
17. A. O. Wosu and C. C. Ibe, "Use of extracts of Picrallima nitida bark in the treatment of experimental trypanosomiasis: A preliminary study," Journal of Ethnopharmacology 25, 3 (1989): 263–268.
18. S. K. Adesina and J. Reisch, "Amides from Zanthoxylum rubescens," Phytochemistry 28, 3 (1989): 839–842.
19. M. M. Iwu and D. L. Clayman, "Evaluation of the in vitro antimalarial activity of Picralima nitida extracts," Journal of Ethnopharmacology 36, 2 (1992): 133–135.
20. J. M. Agbedahunsi and A. J. Aladesanmi, "Antimicrobial activity of Pleioceras barteri root extract," Fitoterapia 64, 1 (1993): 81.
21. A. Obembe et al., "Anti-psychotic effects and tolerance of crude Rauwolfia vomitoria in Nigerian Psychiatric inpatients," Phytotherapy Research 8 (1994): 218–223.
22. F. Omoruyi et al., "Biochemical effects of some local medicinal herbs in rats," Nigerian Journal of Physiological Science 11 (1995): 53–55.
23. A. K. Etu, J. M. Oke, and R. A. Elegbe, "Anti-inflammatory and anti-nociceptive activities from chloroform extract of Voacanga Africana leaf," African Journal of Biomedical Research 4 (2001): 93–96.
24. M. O. Owonubi, E. O. Iwalewa, and M. Shok, "Cardio-activity of Sarmentocide-A from Strophantus sarmentosus seeds," Nigerian J. of Natural Products and Medicine 1, 1 (1997): 16–18.

25. S. I. Inya-agha, "The hypoglycaemic properties of Picralima nitida," Nigerian J. of Natural Products and Medicine 3 (1999): 66–67.

26. C. A. Omenka, "Medical values of Alsonia boonei," Proceedings of the 10th Annual Conference of the BOSUN (Botanical Society of Nigeria) AO16 (1999).

27. O. O. Amole and A. O. Onabanjo, "Antipyretic effect of Rauwolfia vomitoria in rabbits," Nigerian Journal of Natural Products and Medicine 3 (1999): 77–78.

28. L. Costa-Campos et al., "Antipsycotic profile of Alstonine: Ethnopharmacology of a Nigerian botanical remedy," Animal Academy of Bras Cienc 71, 2 (1999): 189–201.

29. L. O. Mgbojikwe and Z. S. C. Okoye, "Acaridicidal efficacy of the aqueous stem bark extract of Adenium obesum on the various life stages of cattle ticks," Nigerian Journal of Experimental Applied Biology 2, 1 (2001): 39–43.

30. M. I. Okeke et al., "Evaluation of extracts of the root of Landolphia owerrience for antibacterial activity," Journal of Ethnopharmacology 78, 2–3 (2001): 119–127.

31. T. O. Fakeye, O. A. Itiola, and H. A. Odelola, "Evaluation of the anti-microbial property of the stem bark of Picralima nitida (Apocynaceae)," Phytotherapy Research 14 (2002): 368–370.

32. T. O. Fakeye et al., "Evaluation of toxicity profile of an alkaloid fraction of the stem bark of Picralima nitida (Family Apocynaceae)," Journal of Herbal Pharmacotherapy (2003).

33. L. Coasta-Campos, M. Iwu, and E. Elisabetsky, "Lack of proconvulsant activity of the antipsychotic alkaloid alstonine," Journal of Ethnopharmacology 93, 2–3 (2004): 307–310.

34. L. Coasta-Campos et al., "Anxiolytic properties of the antipsychotic alkaloid alstonine," Pharmacology, Biochemistry and Behaviour 77, 3 (2004): 481–489.

35. Ibid.

CHAPTER 10

Pharmacological and Physiological Effects Manifested by Twenty Medicinal Plants from Various Botanical Families

Abstract

N MAMMALS, THE renal adjustments of the interstitial fluid to the presence of excess alkali or acids is one of the essential mechanisms the body uses to maintain homeostasis. Possession of diuretic property was therefore regarded as an important attribute of a plant extract and was used to select twenty plants on which this study was done.

This study reviewed and classified the taxonomic family of the plants; the chemical constituents and reported pharmacological effects of the plants and parts of the plant employed in folk medicine based on Ghana Herbal pharmacopeia and various research studies. The results of the study showed that each of the twenty medicinal plants had diuretic effects and several other physiological and pharmacological effects on the body, which included three or more of the following: anti-hypertensive and cardiotonic effects; liver-protective and heart-protective effects; anti-inflammatory effects; hypoglycaemic effects; anti-asthmatic effects; anti-inflammatory, analgesic, and/or antipyretic effects; antimicrobial, antiparasitic, and vermifuge effects; anticancer effects, etc. The plants whose extracts showed a wide range of health-protective effects were *Vernonia amygdalina*, *Bridelia ferruginea*, and *Nauclea latifolia*, and these effects included hypoglycaemic, antihypertensive, liver-protective, lung-protective, anti-inflammatory, analgesic, antipyretic, antimicrobial, and antiparasitic effects. The plant extracts that did not have protective effects on the heart and the cardiovascular system included *Cassia alata*, *Desmodium adscendens*, *Dissotis rotundifolia*, *Huslundia opposite*, *Heliotropium indicum*, *Cola nitida*, *Cymbopogon citrates*, *Cassia podocarpa*, *Trema orientalis*, *Triclisia dictyophylla*, and *Xylopia aethiopica* extracts. The only plant whose extracts produced central nervous system stimulant effects was *Cola nitida*.

These results show that diuretic property can be possessed by medicinal extracts from plants of widely varying taxonomic families and yet these extracts of these various plants will not produce exactly the same pharmacological effects in other organs of the same organism to which they are administered.

Keywords: *diuretic, plant extracts, pharmacological, medicinal, organ-protective, cardio-tonic, effects.*

Introduction

Normal cell function depends on the constancy of the interstitial component of the extracellular fluid, which bathes the body cells. Diuretics increase the net renal excretion of solute and water by inhibiting some of the transport processes the nephron utilizes to reabsorb some of the substances in the glomerular filtrate (which the body still needs) at various sites along the nephron.

Several extracts of plants of varying taxonomic families were reported to have diuretic properties by *Ghana Herbal Pharmacopoeia*.

Although diuretics remain the cornerstone for the treatment of edema or volume overload especially that due to heart failure, ascites, chronic renal failure, and nephrotic syndrome, the use of most currently available diuretics is associated with some problems like disturbing potassium balance which may induce other distressing health conditions. For example, the thiazide diuretics though useful in hypertensive patients with congestive heart failure have the disadvantage of induction of hypokalemic alkalosis, occasional hyperglycemia, and hyperuricemia. The quest for diuretics that give better results is ongoing and justified in this study.

A large number of medicinal plant extracts seem to have diuretic properties. The discovery of diuretic herbal drugs that have a variety of beneficial pharmacologic effects may provide a wider choice of suitable diuretics to choose from in the management of edema and volume overload associated with heart failure and renal failure.

This paper reviews the taxonomical families of twenty diuretic plants; the parts of these plants employed in herbal medicine; the chemical constituents of the extracts of these medicinal plants and the pharmacological characteristics these twenty plants possess other than diuretic activity.

Materials and Methods

Data was generated on the characteristics and pharmacological actions of extracts of twenty medicinal plants of various botanical families identified in *Ghana Herbal Pharmacopoeia*[1] as producing diuretic effects in folklore use and scientific researches as well as from a variety of human and animal studies data.[2–77]

Results

The data on the characteristics and pharmacological actions of twenty diuretic plants of various botanical families generated from information on them in *Ghana Herbal Pharmacopoeia* and a variety of human and animal studies data[2–77] are as shown in tables 1 and 2 below.

Table 1. Twenty medicinal plants, their family, their parts used for herbal medicine, their chemical constituents, and whether or not they have diuretic properties.

Name of Medicinal Plant	Family to Which the Plant Belongs	Plant Parts Used for Medicine	Chemical Constituents of Plant Extract	Diuretic Property
Cassia alata	Caesalpinaceae/Fabaceae	Leaf, flower, seed, root	Tannin, mucillage, anthracene derivatives, free antraquinones (crysophanic acid anthrone), anthraquinone, glycosides (sennosides, rhein)	Present
Vernonia amygdalina	*Asteraceae*	Leaf, roots	Glycosides, tannins, saponins, (vernoniosides), sesquiterpene lactones (vernodaline, vernomygdine, elamanolide), flavonoides (leuteolins), vitamin C	Present
Bridelia ferruginea	Euphorbiaceae	Leaf, stem bark, root bark	Triterpenoids, ligans, eromosele, flavonoids (quercetin, quercetrin, myricitrin, myricetin-3-β-glucoside, ferrugin), biflavanol (gallocatechin-[4-O-7]-epigallocatechin), phenols and tannins.	Present
Combretum smeathmanni	Combretaceae	Leaf, roots	Glycosides, tannins (combretum-cathechin), flavonoids, vitexine, saponaretine, quarternary alkaloids, betaine and choline, organic acids (mallic, glycolic, and glyceric), and potassium nitrate	Present
Desmodium adscendens	Paplionaceae	Aerial parts	Alkaloids, β-phenylethylamine derivatives, N-N-dimethyltryptamine, salsoline, saponins, soyasaponin 1 and 111, soyasapogenol B and E, and cardiac glycosides	Present
Dissotis rotundifolia	Melastomataceae	Leaf, shoot, roots	Reducing sugars, condensed tannins, manganese	Present
Hoslundia opposite Vahl	Labiatae	Leaf, flower, root	Reducing sugars, glycosides, sesquiterpenes (germacrene, β-caryophyiline), and tannins	Present
Heliotropium indicum	Boranginaceae	Leaf, stem, roots, fruits, seeds	Reducing sugars, hydrolyzable tannins and alkaloids (pyrrolizidine alkaloids and their N-oxides [indicine, echinatine, lasiocarpine, indicine N-Oxide, losiocarpine N-Oxide])	Present

Cola nitida	*Sterculiaceae*	Cotyledon, stem bark	Purine alkaloids (caffeine, theobromine), glycosides, (+)- catechin, (-)-epicatechin, phenolics, kolatin, colatein, catechols, and anthocyanins	Present
Cymbopogon citrates DC	Gramineae	Leaves, flowers	Flavonoids and volatile oils (citral, geraniol, citronellal, camphene, and related monoterpenes, triterpenes, and sesquiterpenes)	Present
Lippia multiflora	Verbenaceae	Leaves, stem, roots, fruits, seeds	Flavonoids (glycosides), saponins and volatile oils (linalool, camphor, terpineol, thymol, and other monoterpenes)	Present
Nauclea latifolia	Rubiaceae	Root, leaf, fruit, stem bark	Reducing sugars, tannins, glycoalkaloids and indoloquinolizidines (naucletine, nauclefidine, etc), resins, bitter principles	Present
Cassia occidentalis	Caesalpinaceae	Seeds, leaves, roots	Anthracene glycosides and anthraquinones (sennosides A, B, C; aloe-emodin, etc.), triterpenoids, tannins, flavonoids, fixed oil, toxalbumin (destroyed by roasting)	Present
Phyllantus fratenus	Euphorbiaceae	Leaf	Alkaloids (securinine and related alkaloids), flavonoids (quercetin, rutin, etc), saponins, ligans (phyllantine, hypophyllantine, etc.), carboxylic acid, and methyl salicylate	Present
Cassia podocarpa	Caesalpinaceae	Dried leaflets, roots	Anthracene glycosides, O and C-anthraquinone glycosides, free anthraquinones (emodin)	Present
Solanum torvum	*Solanaceae*	Fruit, leaves, stem, roots	Flavonoids, saponins (glycosides of torvogenin, chlorogenin, sisalagenone), fixed oil, steroidal alkaloids (solasodine, solasonine), coumarins (scopoletin, scopolin, aesculin), vitamin B stoup, vitamin C and iron salts, β-sitosterol	Present
Trema orientalis	Ulmaceae	Leaf, heartwood, bark	Triterpenods (simiarenol, trematol, and related triterpenes), tannins, volatile oil, lupeol, -(-)epicatechin, scopoletin, *p*-hydroxybenzoic acid, and reducing sugars	Present

Triclisia dictyophylla	Menispermaceae	Whole plant	Alkaloids; phaenthine; trigilletine, stebisimine, cosculine, isotetrandrine, triclisine, tricliseine, inositol	present
Xylopia aethiopica	*Annonaceae*	Fruits, stem bark, root bark	Oleoresins, volatile oils (monoterpenoids, cineole, cuminic aldehyde, terpinone, β-pinene), diterpenoids (xylopic acid, other kaurane, trachylobane, and kolavane diterpenoids), minerals (copper, manganese and zinc)	Present
Momordica charanthia	*Cucurbitaceae*	Aerial parts, fruit, seed, whole plant	Alkaloid (momordicine), fatty acid, charantin, γ-aminobutyric acid, volatile oil, vitamin C, carotenoids (cryptoxanthin, β-carotene, cucurbitacins, saponins, rosmarinic acid, and carbohydrates	-

Table 2. Pharmacologic, medicinal, and organ effects of the twenty diuretic plants.

Name of Plant	Effects on Pain, Inflammation, and Fever	Organ-Protective Effects	Other Effects	Effects on Infective Organisms
Cassia alata	Febrifuge effects	Hypoglycaemic effects	Choloretic, purgative, laxative, digestive effects	Antibacterial, antifungal, insecticidal/ repellant effects
Vernonia amygdalina	Analgesic, anti-inflammatory, antipyretic, antirheumatic effects	Liver- and heart-protective, antioxidant, antihypertensive, body-calming/sedative, anticancer/ antitumor,nti-tumor and hypoglycaemic effects	Blood expander, anti-obesity (lipid-lowering), wound-healing, anticatarrhal, pro-fertility, mucolytic; bronchodilator, anti-anaphylactic, anti-aging, immune-stimulant effects	Antimicrobial, antifungal, antimalarial, antihelminthic, anti-leishmaniasis, insect-repellant effects
Bridelia ferruginea	Anti-inflammatory effects	Antihypertensive, Antitumor, hypoglycaemic effects	Anti-anaphylactic, Antispasmodic effects	Antimicrobial, antifungal, antiviral, Antihelminthic effects

Combretum *smeathmannii*	Anti-inflammatory, antipyretic, antirheumatic effects	Liver- protective, Slight antihypertensive effects	Vulnerary, choleretic, cholagogue effects	Antiviral, antimicrobial, antihelminthic effects
Desmodium adscendens	Analgesic, anti-inflammatory, and antipyretic effects	Bronchodilator, galactogogue, anticonvulsant /antiepileptic effects.	Anti-asthmatic, Anti-anaphylactic, Anti-histamine, Muscle-relaxant (antispasmodic), vulnerary effects	
Dissotis rotundifolia	Anti-inflammatory, and antipyretic effects		Anti-asthmatic effects	Antimicrobial effects
Hoslundia opposite	Analgesic, anti-inflammatory, and antipyretic effects.	CNS depressant, sedative, anticonvulsant effects		Antimicrobial, antimalarial effects
Heliotropium indicum	Anti-inflammatory effects			Antibacterial, Antihelminthic, antifungal
Cola nitida		CNS stimulant, Anti-depressant Effects.		
Cymbopogon citrates	Analgesic, anti-inflammatory, antipyretic; antirheumatic effects			Antifungal, insect-repellant effects
Lippia multiflora	Analgesic effects	Antihypertensive, tranquilizing effects	Laxative, sudorific, muscle-relaxant effects	Antimicrobial, antimalarial, insect-repellant effects
Nauclea latifolia	Antipyretic effects	Liver-protective, antihypertensive anticancer (cytotoxic), hypoglycaemic effects	Anti-hemorrhoids, stomachic, toner, body-calming effects	Antibacterial, antimalarial, antitrypanasome, antiparasitic, antifungal, antihelminthic effects

Cassia occidentalis	Antipyretic effects	Liver-protective, organ-protective, antihypertensive, antimutagenic effects	Laxative, purgative, cholagouge, abortifacient effects	Antimicrobial, mild antimalarial effect, Antiparasitic effects
Phyllantus fraternus	Analgesic, Anti-inflammatory, and antipyretic effects	Liver-protective, Antihypertensive, antimutagenic, hypoglycaemic effects	Tonic, antispasmodic, laxative, stomachic, choleratic; carminative, digestive effects	Antiviral; antibacterial; antiprotozoal, antimalarial, and vermifuge effects
Cassia podocarpa			Laxative and/or purgative effects.	
Solanum torvum		Sedative, moderate anticonvulsant, carditonic, hemantic, hemostatic (postpartum) effects	Vulnerary, Vulnerary, Digestive, tonic effects	Antimicrobial, fungistatic effects
Trema orientalis	Analgesic, Anti-inflammatory, and antipyretic effects	Anticonvulsant, hypoglycaemic effects	Antituisive effects.	Antimicrobial, antibacterial, antihelminthic effects
Triclisia dictyophylla	Anti-inflammatory, antipyretic, anti-edematous, anti-arthritic effects	Hemantic, anticancer effects	Antispasmodic effects	Antimicrobial, antimalarial, antiprotozoal, Antitrypanosome, and anti-leishmaniasis effects
Xylopia aethiopica	Anti-inflammatory; antipyretic effects		Stimulant, carminative, postpartum tonic, lactation aid, lipid-lowering, and antispasmodic effects	Anti-bacterial; Anti-fungal; Broad spectrum anti-biotic Effects.
Momordica charantia	Anti-inflammatory, febrifuge effects	Antidiabetic; anti-ulcer; antitumor, antineoplastic, antioxidant effects	Antifertility, astringent, vulnerary effects	Antimicrobial, antiviral, antihelminthic effects

The diuretic plant extracts that produced antihypertensive and cardiotonic effects are *Vernonia amygdalina*, *Bridelia ferruginea*, *Combretum smeathmanni*, *Lippia grandifolia*, *Nauclea latifolia*, *Cassia occidentalis*, *Phyllantus fratenus*, and *Solanum torvum*. The diuretic plant extracts that were shown here to have liver- and heart-protective properties are *Vernonia amygdalina*, *Combretum smeathmanni*, *Cassia occidentalis*, and *Phyllantus fratenus* extracts. The plant extracts that produced anti-inflammatory properties are *Vernonia amygdalina*, *Bridelia ferruginea*, *Combretum smeathmanni*, *Desmodium adscendens*, *Dissotis rotundifolia*, *Huslundia opposite*, *Heliotropium indicum*, *Cymbopogon citrates*, *Triclisia dictyophylla*, *Phyllantus fratenus*, *Trema orientalis*, and *Xylopia aethiopica* extracts. The plant extracts which did not have protective effects on the heart and the cardiovascular system included *Cassia alata*, *Desmodium adscendens*, *Dissotis rotundifolia*, *Huslundia opposite*, *Heliotropium indicum*, *Cola nitida*, *Cymbopogon citrates*, *Cassia podocarpa*, *Trema orientalis*, *Triclisia dictyophylla*, and *Xylopia aethiopica* extracts. Of particular note is *Cola nitida* extract which produced central nervous system stimulant effects only. The plants whose extracts showed a wide range of health-protective effects were *Vernonia amygdalina*, *Bridelia ferruginea*, and *Nauclea latifolia*. These protective effects included hypoglycaemic, antihypertensive, liver-protective, lung-protective, anti-inflammatory, analgesic, antipyretic, antimicrobial, antiparasitic, antioxidant/lipolytic, antispasmodic, and anticancer effects.

Discussions

Since diuretics are often employed in the treatment of edema or volume overload especially that due to heart failure, ascites, chronic renal failure, and nephrotic syndrome, diuretic plant extracts which also produce antihypertensive and cardiotonic or heart-protective effects may with more refinement contribute to effective treatment of hypertension and heart failure.

The diuretic plant extracts which in this study were reported to also produce antihypertensive and cardiotonic effects are *Vernonia amygdalina*, *Bridelia ferruginea*, *Combretum smeathmanni*, *Lippia grandifolia*, *Nauclea latifolia*, *Cassia occidentalis*, *Phyllantus fratenus*, and *Solanum torvum* while those shown to have liver- and heart-protective properties are *Vernonia amygdalina*, *Combretum smeathmanni*, *Cassia occidentalis*, and *Phyllantus fratenus* extracts. On the other hand, the plant extracts which did not have protective effects on the heart and the cardiovascular system included *Cassia alata*, *Desmodium adscendens*, *Dissotis rotundifolia*, *Huslundia opposite*, *Heliotropium indicum*, *Cola nitida*, *Cymbopogon citrates*, *Cassia podocarpa*, *Trema orientalis*, *Triclisia dictyophylla*, and *Xylopia aethiopica* extract. *Cola nitida* was so different from the other nineteen plants examined that it alone had central nervous system stimulant effects and no other effects, which points to the danger to the brain and other organs of the body of consumption of high doses of *Cola nitida*.

Many diseases, health disorders, and accidental physiological traumas and insults that affect the body are associated with inflammation and pain, suggesting the importance of the plant extracts in this study that have analgesic, antipyretic, and anti-inflammatory properties. The plant extracts which have these properties included *Vernonia amygdalina*, *Bridelia ferruginea*, *Combretum smeathmanni*, *Desmodium adscendens*, *Dissotis rotundifolia*, *Huslundia opposite*, *Heliotropium indicum*, *Cymbopogon citrates*, *Triclisia dictyophylla*, *Phyllantus fratenus*, *Trema orientalis*, and *Xylopia aethiopica* extracts.

Of the twenty diuretic plant extracts, only extracts of *Vernonia amygdalina*, *Bridelia ferruginea*, and *Nauclea latifolia* have the following wide-range beneficial effects: hypoglycaemic, antihypertensive, liver-protective, lung-protective, anti-inflammatory, analgesic, antipyretic, antimicrobial, and antiparasitic effects.

Conclusions

The findings of this study suggest that diuretic property can be possessed by medicinal extracts from plants of widely varying taxonomic families, yet the extracts of these diuretic plants will have widely different effects on different parts of the body reflective of the properties of the plant families to which the individual plants belong. The findings of this study also suggest that extracts of plants which besides diuretic effects, produce antihypertensive, cardiotonic, liver-protective, anti-inflammatory, and heart-protective effects in the body like *Vernonia amygdalina*, *Bridelia ferruginea*, *Combretum smeathmanni*, *Lippia multiflora*, *Nauclea latifolia*, *Cassia occidentalis*, *Phyllantus fratenus*, *Cassia occidentalis*, and *Solanum torvum* may, in future when improved upon, prove to be of assistance as adjuncts in relief of edema and volume overload associated with some cardiovascular and renal disorders.

References

1. Kofi Busia, ed., Ghana Herbal Pharmacopoeia (Accra, Ghana: Science and Technology Policy Research Institute, 2007).
2. B. A. Iwalokun et al., "Hepato-protective and Antioxidant Activity of Vernonia amygdalina on Acetoaminophen-Induced Hepatic Damage in Mice," J. of Medicinal Food 9, 4 (2006): 524–530.
3. A. Aroka et al., "Analgesic, Anti-plasmodial Activity and Toxicology of Vernonia amygdalina," Journal of Medicinal Food 11, 3 (2008): 574–581.
4. Uchechukwu Anastasia Utoh-Nedosa and Nedosa Ebelechukwu Eleanor, "Sleep Producing Effect of Vernonia amygdalina Leaf Extract in Humans: It's Associated Factors," Inventi Rapid: Molecular Pharmacology 2012, no. 1 (April 12, 2011).
5. Research Journal of Medicinal Sciences, "Anti-inflammatory Activity of Ethanolic Extract from Vernonia amygdalina on the Immune System of Swiss Albino Rats," Research J. of Medicinal Scs. 1, 2 (2007): 127–131.
6. H. U. Nwanjo, "Efficacy of aqueous leaf extract of Vernonia amygdalina on plasma lipoprotein and oxidative status in diabetic rat models," Nigerian Journal of Physiological Sciences 20, no. 1 (2005).
7. M. Jisaka et al., "Anti-tumoral and Antimicrobial Activities of Bitter Sesquiterpene Lactones of Vernonia amygdalina, a possible medicinal Plant Used by Chimpanzees," Bioscience, Biotechnology, Biochemistry 57, 5 (1993): 833–834.
8. B. A. Iwalokun et al., "Hepatoprotective and Antioxidant Activity of Vernonia amygdalina on Acetoaminophen-Induced Hepatic Damage in Mice," Journal of Medicinal Food 9, 4 (2006): 524–530.
9. C. F. Anowi et al., "The Antimicrobial Activity of the Crude Extract of Vernonia amygdalina del (Asteraceae) Leaf," IJPI's Journal of Pharmacognosy and Herbal Formulations (2011), www.ijpijournals.com.
10. A. Tadesse, A. Gebre-Hiwot, and K. Asres, "In vitro activity of Vernonia amygdalina on Leishmania aethiopica," Ethiop. Med. J. 31, 3 (1993): 183–189.

11. Index Medicus Afro WHO, "The Wound Healing Effects of Herbal Ointments Formulated with Leaves of Vernonia amygdalina Var" (2009), indexmedicus.afro.who.int/iah/fulltex/jophas3.7esimone.pdf-lignende http://www 7/4/2009.

12. I. Addae-Mensah and R. W. Munenge, "Quercetin-3-neohesperidose (rutin) and other flavonoids as the active hypoglycaemic agents in Bridelia ferruginea," Fitoterapia 10, 4 (1989): 359–362.

13. Mocol 79, 2: 249–251.

14. O. A. Olajide, J. M. Makinde, and S. O. Awe, "Effects of the Aqueous Extract of Bridlia ferruginea Stem Bark on Carreginaan-induced Oedema and Granuloma tissue formation in Rats and Mice," J. Ethnopharmacol 66, 1 (1999): 113–117.

15. K. Cimanga et al., "Radical Scavenging and xanthine oxidase inhibitory activity of phenolic compounds from Bridelia ferruginea" (2001).

16. O. Onoruvwe et al., "Effects of Stem Bark and Leaf extracts of Bridelia ferruginea on Rat Bladder Smooth Muscle," Fitoterapia 72, 3 (2001): 230–236.

17. D. A. Akinpelu and F. O. Olorunmola, Antimicrobial activity of Bridelia ferruginea Fruit," Fititherapia 71 (2000): 75–76.

18. A. O. Olajide, D. T. Okpako, and J. M. Makinde, "Anti-inflammatory properties of Bridelia ferruginea Stem Bark, Inhibition of lipopolysaccharide-induced Septic Shock and Vascular permeability," J. of Ethnophamacol. 82, 2–3 (2003): 221–224.

19. O. Onoruvwe et al., "Effects of Stem Bark and Leaf extracts of Bridelia ferruginea on Skeletal Muscle," Phytother. Res. 8 (1994): 38–41.

20. M. E. Addy and W. K. Dzandu, "Dose-response Effects of Desmodium adscendens aqueous extract on histamine response, content and anaphylactic Reaction in the Guinea pig," J. Ethnopharmacol 18, 1 (1986): 13–20.

21. P. Nguemo, Baldy Moulinier, and Bina C. Nguemby, "Effects of an ethanolic extract of Desmodium adscendens on Central Nervous System in Rodents," J. Ethnopharmacol 52, 2 (1966): 77–83.

22. O. A. Olajide, S. O. Awe, and J. M. Makinde, "Central Nervous System Depressant Effect of Hoslundia opposite Vahl," Phytother. Res. 13, 5 (1999): 425–426.

23. G. M. Gundidza et al., "Antimicrobial Activity of essential oil from Huslundia opposite," Cent. Afr. J. Med. 38, 7 (1992): 290–293.

24. R. J. Suresh, R. P. Rajeswara, and M. S. Reddy, "Wound Healing Effects of Helitropium indicum, Plumbago zeylanicum, and Acalypha indica in Rats. J. Ethnopharmacol. 79, 2 (2002): 249–251.

25. K. Srinivas, M. E. B. Rao, and S. S. Rao, "Anti-inflammatory activity of Helitropium indicum Linn and Leucas aspera spreng in albino Rats," Indian J. Pharmacol. 32, 1 (2000): 37–38.

26. R. Trindal, "The culture of Cola: Social and Economic Aspects of a West Arical Domesticate," in Ethnobotanical Leaflets (Carbondale: Southern Illinois University Hebarium, 1997).

27. B. Wannissom, S. Jarikasen, and T. Soontoanasart, "Anti-fungal Activity of Lemon Grass Oils and Lemon Grass Oil Cream," Physiother. Res. 10 (1996): 551–554.

28. B. B. Lorenzetti, G. E. P. Souza, and S. J. Sarti, "Myrcene Mimics the Peripheral Analgesic Activity of Lemon Grass Tea," J. EthnoPharmacol 34 (1991): 43–48.

29. E. O. Lima et al., "In-vitro Anti-fungal Activity of Essential Oils obtained from Officinal Plants against Dermatophytes," Mycoses 36, 910 (1993): 333–336.

30. O. Kunle et al., "Antimicrobial Activity of Various Extracts and Carvacrol from Lippia multilora Leaf Extract," Phytomed. 10, 1 (2003): 59–61.

31. A. A. Abenna, G. R. Ngondzo-Kombeti, and D. Bioka, "Psychopharmacologic Properties of Lippia multiflora," 31. Article in French, Encephale. 24, 5 (1998): 449–454.

32. Pham Huu Chanh, K. Yao, and A. Pham Huu Chann, "Comparative Hypotensive Effects of Compounds Extracted from Lippia multiflora Leaves," Planta Med. 54 (1988): 294–296.

33. J. W. Mwangi et al., "Essential Oils of Lippia spp. in Kenya IV, Maize weevil (Sitophlus zeamais) Repellency and Larvicidal Activity," Intern J. Crude Drug Res. (1991).

34. A. Gidado, D. A. Amen, and S. E. Atawodi, "Effect of Nauclea latifolia Aqueous Leaf Extract on Blood Glucose Levels of Normal and Alloxan-induced Diabetic Rats," Africa Journal of Biotech. 4, 1 (2005): 91–93.

35. S. Amos et al., "Neuropharmacological Effects of the Aqueous Extract of Nauclea latifolia Root Bark in Rats and Mice," J. Ethnopharmacol. 10, 97, 1 (2005): 53–57.

36. P. A. Onyeyili et al., "Antihelmintic Activity of Crude Aqueous Extract of Nauclea latifolia Stem Bark Against Ovine Nematodes," Fitoterapia 72, 1 (2001): 12–21.

37. I. I. Madubunyi, "Anti-Hepatotoxic and Trypanocidal Activities of the Ethanolic Extract of Nauclea latifolia Root Bark," J. Herbs Spices Med. Plants 3, 2 (1995): 23–53.

38. Y. Deeni and H. Hussain, "Screening for Antimicrobial Activity and for Alkaloids of Nauclea latifolia," J. Ethnopharmacol 35 (1991): 91–96.

39. "Immunomodulatory Properties of Vernonia amygdalina Extract in Swiss Albino Rats" (2007), medwelljournals.com/fulltext/rjms/2007/127-131.pdf.

40. "Lignende efter M Oladunmoye-Relaterede artikler," medwelljournals-Alle 2 versioner http://www 7/4/2009.

41. P. A. Akah and C. L. Okafor, "Blood Sugar-Lowering Effects of Vernonia amygdalina Del in an experimental Rabbit Model," Phytotherapy Research 6, no. 3 (2006): 171–173.

42. The Free Library, "Overview of Divisional Programs," www.thefreelibrary.com/Overview+of+Divisional+Programs.-a0176375431.

43. D. N. Siamba et al., "Efficacy of Tephrosa vogelli and Vernonia amygdalina as Anti-helminthics against Ascaridia galli in Indigenous Chicken," Lifestock Research for Rural Development 19, 12 (2007).

44. D. A. Alabi, L. A. Jimoh Oyero, and N. A. B. Amusa, "Fungitoxic and Phytotoxic Effects of Vernonia amygdalina, Bryophyllum pinnatus Kurtz, Ocimum gratissimum (Closium) and Eucalyptus globules (Caliptos) Labile Water Extracts on Cowpea Seedlings in Ago-Iwoye, Southwestern Nigeria," Journal of Agricultural Science 1, 1 (2005).

45. Uchechukwu Anastasia Utoh-Nedosa, "Normal Hair Colour, Hair Texture, Hair Form, Hair Lusture and Hair Condition Restoration Effects of Aqueous Vernonia amygdalina Leaf Extract," Inventi Rapid: Cosmeceuticals 2011, no. 3 (2011).

46. Uchechukwu Anastasia Utoh-Nedosa, "Wound Healing; Antimicrobial; Analgesic; Anti-inflammatory and Immune Defence Effects of Vernonia amygdalina Aqueous Leaf Extract, and Leaf Powder In Vivo," Inventi Rapid: Planta Activa 2011, no. 1 (2011).

47. Uchechukwu Anastasia Utoh-Nedosa et al., "Excess Body Fat Elimination (Anti-Obesity) Effects of Vernonia Amygdalina Leaf Extract," American Journal of Pharmacology and Toxicology 6, 2 (2011): 55–58.

48. Uchechukwu Utoh-Nedosa, "The Body Calming And Body Vitalizing Effects of Vernonia amygdalina Leaf Extract and Leaf Powder and Their Mechanisms," American Journal of Agriculture and Biological Sciences 6, 3 (2011): 429–432.

49. Uchechukwu Utoh-Nedosa, "Anti-Carcinoma, Anti-Obesity, Antidiabetic and Immune Defence Effects of Vernonia amygdalina Leaf Extract and Leaf Powder, in Two Human Cancer Patients," American Journal of Immunology 6, 4 (2010): 50–53.

50. Uchechukwu Anastasia Utoh-Nedosa, "The External Anti-aging Effects of Vernonia amygdalina Leaf Extract on the Human Body and the Effect of Protein Intake, Carbohydrate Intake and the Weather on Them," Inventi Rapid: Molecular Pharmacology 2011, no. 4 (2011).

51. 73.R. O. Akomolafe et al., "An in-vitro Study of the Effects of Cassia podocarpa Fruit on the Intestinal Motility of Rats," Phytomed. 11, 2–3 (2004): 249–54.

52. S. K. Adesina, "Studies on some Plants Used As Anti-convulsants in Amerindian and African Traditional Medicine," Fitoterapia, (1982): 147–162.

53. W. W. A. Bergers and G. M. Alink, "Toxic Effects of Glucoalkaloids Solanine and Tomatine on Cultured Neonatal Rat Heart Cells," Toxicol. Letters 6 (1980): 29–32.

54. N. Sharma et al., "Protective Effects of Cassia occidentalis on Chemical-Induced Chromosomal Aberrations in Mice," Ann. Trop. Medicine and Parasitol. 95, 1 (2001): 47–57.

55. P. P. Rai and M. Shok, "Anthraquinone Glycosides from Plant Parts of Cassia occidentalis," Indian J. Chem. 45 (1983): 87–88.

56. M. Gasquet et al., "Evaluation In-vitro and In-vivo of a Traditional Antimalarial, 'Malaria 5,'" Fitoterapia 64 (1993): 423–426.

57. P. J. O'Hara and K. R. Pierce, "Toxic Cardio-myopathy caused by Cassia occidentals in Poisoned Rabbits," Vet Pathol. 11 (1974): 110–124.

58. L. Tona et al., "In-vivo Antimalarial Activity of Cassia ocidentalis, Morinda morindoides and Phyllantus niruri," Drug Chem. Toxicol 22, 4 (1999): 643–653.

59. A. A. Chowdhury and M. S. Islam, "Anti-microbial Activity of Trema orientalis," Dhaka University J. Pharmaceut. Sci. 3 (2004): 1–2.

60. R. Barbear et al., "Analgesic and Anti-inflammatory Activity in Acute and Chronic Conditions of Trema guieense Shum & Thonn) Ficalho and T. Michrantha Blume Extracts in Rodents," Phytother Res. 6 (1992): 146–148.

61. T. Dimo et al., "Glucose Lowering Efficacy of the Steh Bark Extract of Trema orientalis (linn) Blume, in Normal and Streptozotocin Diabetic Rats," Pharmazie 61, 3 (2006): 233–236.

62. E. H. Herman and D. P. Chadwick, "Cardiovascular Effects of D-Tetrandine," Pharmacol. 12 (1974): 97–109.

63. A. I. Spiff et al., "Constituents of West African Medicinal Plant, 30, Tridictyophylline, a New Morphine-like alkaloid from Triclisia dictyophylla," J. Nat. Prod. 44 (1981): 160–165.

64. L. I. Somova et al., "Cardiovascular and Diuretic Activity of Kaurene Derivatives of Xylopia aethiopica and Alepidea amatymbica," Ethnopharmacol. 77, 2–3 (2001): 165–174.

65. L. N. Tatsadjieu et al., "Anti-bacterial and Anti-fungal Activity of Xylopia aethiopica, Monodra myristica, Zanthozyllum xanthoxyloides and Zanthoxylum lepieurii from Cameroon," Fitoterapia 74, 5 (2003): 469–472.

66. K. Boakye-Yiadom, N. Fiagbe, and S. Ayim, "Anti-microbial Properties of Some West African Plants IV. Antimicrobial Activity of Xylopic acid and some other Constituents of the Fruit of Xylopia aethiopica (Annonaceae)," Lloydia 40, 6 (1977): 543–545.

67. S. A. Igwe, J. C. Afonne, and S. I. Ghasic, "Ocular Dynamics of Systemic Aqueous Extracts of Xylopia aethiopica (African Guinea pepper) Seeds on Visually Active Volunteers," J. of Ethnophamacol. 86, 2–3 (2003): 139–142.

68. B. Ahmed, T. A. al-Howiriny, and R. Mathew, "Anti-hepatotoxic Activity of Phyllantus fratenus," Pharmazie 57, 12 (2000): 855–856.

69. V. I. Hukeri, "Hypoglycaemic Activity of Flavonoids of Phyllantu niruri in Rats," Fitoterapia 59, 1 (1988): 68–70.

70. A. H. Campos, "Phyllanthus niruri Inhibits Calcium Oxalate Endocytosis by Renal Tubular Cells: Its Role in Urolithiasis," Nephron 81, 4 (1999): 393–397.

71. C. R. Hung, "Prophylactic Effects of Sucralfate and Geranin on Ethanol-Induced gastric mucosal Damage in Rats," Chin J. Physiol 38, 4 (1995): 211–217.

72. A. M. Freitas, "The Effect of Phyllantus niruri on Urinary Inhibitors of Calcium Oxalate Crystallization and other factors associated with Renal Stone Formation," B. J. U. Int. 89, 9 (2002): 829–834.

73. A. R. Santos, "Antinociceptive Properties of Extracts of New Species of Plants of the Genus Phyllantus (Euphorbiaceae)," J. Ethnopharmacol 72, 1/2 (2000): 229–238.

74. L. Ogata, "HIV-1 reverse transcriptase inhibitor from Phyllantus niruri," AIDS Res Hum Retroviruses 8, 11 (1992): 1937–1944.

75. H. Ueno, "Chemical and Pharmaceutical Studies on Medicinal Plants in Paraguay, Geranin, an Angiotensin-converting Enzyme Inhibitor from 'paraparai mi,' Phyllantus niruri," J. Nat. Prod. 51, 2 (1988): 357–359.

76. M. X. Wang, "Observations of the efficacy of Phyllantus spp. in treating patients with chronic hepatitis B," in Ghana Herbal Pharmacopoeia, ed. Kofi Busia (Accra, Ghana: Science and Technology Policy Research Institute, 1994), 750–752.

77. N. Srividya "Diuretic, Hypotensive and Hypoglycaemic Effects of Phyllantus amarus," J. Indian Exp. Biol. 33, 11 (1995): 861–864.

CHAPTER 11

The Longevity and Stability of the Medicinal Constituents of Plant Extracts and Juices

WHEN PLANT MATERIALS like leaves, stems, stem barks, shoots, flowers, roots, root barks, etc. are dried, moisture that can support the growth of pathogenic organisms is eliminated from them. In the dry state, the medicinally active ingredients in medicinal plants stay active for many years provided that the dry plant materials are stored well in cool, dry, shaded, dark, or dim clean environments. Extracts and juices prepared from fresh plant materials should be made to be concentrated. Plant materials that have a high liquid content should be preferably extracted neatly because the addition of water would dilute and weaken the extract and might expose it to microbial attack. Plant material like citrus fruits should be extracted neatly if they are intended to stay long on the shelf for use. Already prepared medicinal plant materials like those that have been milled, freeze-dried, distilled, etc., can lose some of their pharmacological (medicinal) activity if they are not well corked (tightly covered) or are frequently opened and left open for minutes at a time, especially if they have volatile constituents.

Undue exposure or excessive exposure to light, heat, high pressures, acidity, and other adverse weather conditions can cause already prepared medicinal plant extracts (or the materials from which they are made) to change color or taste or lose some activity or become rancid if they contain oils.

Below is a report of a study that illustrates that if properly stored, some medicinal (herbal) extracts or juices can be pharmacologically active for twenty to fifty or more years. This study is likely to be continued to get more data on the longevity of some of the samples used in this study.

The research report is as follows:

Antimicrobial Screening of Freshly Prepared, Ten-Years-Stored and Twenty-Years-Stored Lime Juices

Materials

Lime Juices

Three different lime juices prepared at different times were used in this study: lime juice 1 (freshly prepared), lime juice 2 (prepared ten years ago), and lime juice 3 (prepared twenty years ago). The lime juices used in this study are shown in figure 1.

Culture Media and Other Reagents Used in the Microbiological Analyses

Nutrient agar, nutrient broth, Mueller-Hinton agar, Sabouraud dextrose agar, Sabouraud dextrose broth (Oxoid UK).

Test Organisms

Four (4) strains of both gram-negative and gram-positive bacteria (*Escherichia coli*, *Salmonella typhi*, *Staphylococcus aureus*, and *Bacillus subtilis*) and two fungal strains (*Aspergillus niger* and *Candida albicans*) were used in this study. These were clinical isolates obtained from the Department of Pharmaceutical Microbiology and Biotechnology, Faculty of Pharmaceutical Sciences, Nnamdi Azikiwe University, Awka.

Methods

Primary Screening of Plant Extract for Antibacterial and Antifungal Activity

The antibacterial and antifungal activities of the fresh, ten-year-old and twenty-year-old lime juices were determined by the agar well diffusion method as described by Perez et al. (1990).

Twenty (20) mL of molten Mueller-Hinton Agar (MHA) and Sabouraud dextrose agar (SDA) (for bacterial and fungal isolates respectively) were poured into sterile petri dishes (90 mm) and allowed to set. Standardized concentrations (McFarland 0.5) of overnight cultures of test isolates were swabbed aseptically on the agar plates and holes (6 mm) were made in the agar plates using a sterile metal cork-borer. Twenty (20 µL) of the various lime juices and controls were put in each hole under aseptic condition, kept at room temperature for 1 hour to allow the agents to diffuse into the agar medium and incubated accordingly. Gentamicin (10 µg/mL) and Fluconazole (25 µg/mL) were used as positive controls in the antibacterial and antifungal evaluations respectively; while sterile distilled water was used as the negative control. The MHA plates were then incubated at 37°C for twenty-four hours, and the SDA plates were incubated at room temperature (25°C–27°C) for two to three days. The inhibition zones diameters (IZDs) were measured and recorded. The size of the cork borer (6 mm) was deducted from the values recorded for the IZDs to get the actual diameter. This procedure was conducted in triplicate and the mean IZDs were calculated and recorded. The experiment was repeated after three months with the same samples.

Table 1. Inhibition zone diameters (IZD) produced by the first antimicrobial evaluation of fresh, ten-year-old and twenty-year-old lime juices on test isolates.

Test Isolates	IZDs (mm)												
	Lime Juice 1 (fresh)				Lime Juice 2 (10 years)				Lime Juice 3 (20 years)				Controls	
													Positive	Negative
	A	B	C	ẋ	A	B	C	ẋ	A	B	C	ẋ	Gentamicin (10 ug)	Water

Escherichia coli E. coli	17	18	18	17	15	15	15	15	10	11	10	10	24	0
Staphylococcus aur S. S aureus S S. S aureus	12	11	11	12	10	10	10	10	6	6	6	6	20	0
Salmonella typhiS	15	16	15	15	15	16	16	16	6	6	5	6	27	0
Bacillus subtilis	12	11	12	12	11	10	10	10	7	7	8	7	24	0
													Fluconazole (50 µg)	Water
Aspergillus niger	0	0	0	0	0	0	0	0	0	0	0	0	15	0
Candida albicans	23	25	23	24	23	23	22	24	15	17	15	16	25	0

ẋ- Mean IZDs

Table 2. Inhibition zone diameters (IZDs) produced by fresh, ten-year-old and twenty-year-old lime juices on test isolates at repeat anti-microbial evaluation after three months of the first evaluation.

Test Isolates	Mean IZDs				
	Lime Juice 1 (fresh)(fresh)	Lime Juice 2 (10 years)(10 years)	Lime Juice 3 (20 years)(20 years)	Controls	
				Positive	Negative
				Gentamicin (10 ug)	Water
E. coli	17	15	10	24	0
Staph. aureus	12	10	6	32	0
S. typhi	15	16	6	23	0
B. Subtilis	12	10	7	34	0
				Fluconazole (50 µg)	
Asper. niger	0		0	8	0
Candida albicans	24	24	7	14	0

Test Isolates	Mean IZDs				
	Lime Juice 1 (fresh)(fresh)	Lime Juice 2 (10 years) (10 years)	Lime Juice 3 (20 years)(20 years)	Controls	
				Positive	Negative
				Gentamicin (10 ug)	Water
Escherichia coli	17	15	10	24	0
Staphylococcus aureus	12	10	6	32	0
Salmonella typhi	15	16	6	23	0
Bacillus subtilis	12	10	7	34	0
				Fluconazole (50 μg)	Water
Aspergillus niger	0	0	0	8	0
Candida albicans	24	24	7	14	0

Results and Discussions

These results obtained clearly demonstrated that lime juice has antibacterial and antifungal properties even when the lime juice is ten years or twenty years old. The antibacterial effects of lime juice were in the order: activity of the lime juices against *Escherichia coli* > *Staphylococcus aureus* > *Salmonella typhi* > *Bacillus subtilis*.

Fresh lime juice, ten-year-old lime juice, and twenty-year-old lime juice produced 75%, 63%, and 42% activity of the anti-*Escherichia-coli* activity of gentamycin respectively. These results show that lime juice has a very strong antibacterial activity against *Escherichia coli* even after ten to twenty years of storage.

The fresh, ten-year-old, and twenty-year-old lime juices demonstrated 60%, 55%, and 30% of the activity of gentamycin respectively against *Staphylococcus aureus*. These results also show that lime juice has a strong activity against Staphylococcus aureus even after ten to twenty years of storage.

The fresh, ten-year-old, and twenty-year-old lime juices produced 56%, 60%, and 23% of the activity of gentamycin respectively against *Salmonella typhi*. These results also show that lime juice has a strong activity against *Salmonella typhi* because even after ten years of storage lime juice produced 60% of the antibacterial effect of gentamycin against *Salmonella typhi*. It is noteworthy however that the anti-*Salmonella-typhi* activity of ten-year-old lime juice was superior to that of fresh lime juice and twenty-year-old lime juice. There must be a substance that is active against *Salmonella typhi* that built up in lime juice while the lime juice was in storage for ten years.

Fresh, ten-year-old, and twenty-year-old lime juices demonstrated 50%, 45.86%, and 31.25% of the activity of gentamycin respectively against *Bacillus subtilis*. These results also show that lime juice has a fairly strong activity against *Bacillus subtilis* even after ten to twenty years of storage.

None of the fresh, ten-year-old, and twenty-year-old lime juices showed activity against *Aspergillus niger* fungus. But the three samples of lime juice demonstrated very high activity against *Candida albicans*. Fresh lime juice elicited 96% of the activity of fluconazole, ten-years-old lime juice elicited 92% of the activity of fluconazole, and twenty-year-old lime juice elicited 64% of the activity of fluconazole. These results suggest that fresh and ten-year-old lime juices have as much antifungal effect against *Candida albicans* as the standard antifungal drug fluconazole. The results also show that even after twenty years of storage, lime juice retains as much as 60% of the antifungal effect of the standard orthodox antifungal drug fluconazole.

The Results of the Repeat Antimicrobial Evaluation of Fresh, Ten-Year-Old, and Twenty-Year-Old Lime Juice Samples Three Months after the First Evaluation

A repeat antimicrobial evaluation of the same samples of fresh, ten-year-old, and twenty-year-old lime juices was done three months after the first antimicrobial evaluation under the same experimental conditions. This repeat antimicrobial evaluation of the three lime juice samples produced the results in table 2.

In these results, fresh lime juice, ten-year-old lime juice, and twenty-year-old lime juice produced 70%, 63%, and 42% of the anti-*Escherichia-coli* activity of gentamycin respectively as against the 75%, 63%, and 45% activity they produced three months earlier. These results demonstrated that after being left on the shelf in the open laboratory for three months, these three samples of lime juice produced a similar high anti-*E. coli* activity as they did three months earlier. It was the anti-*Escherichia-coli* activity of fresh and twenty-year-old lime juice samples that dropped slightly from 75% and 45% to 70% and 42% respectively but the anti-*E. coli* activity of ten-year-old lime juice remained the same.

The results of the repeat evaluation of the antibacterial activity of fresh lime juice, ten-year-old lime juice, and twenty-year-old lime juice after three months against *Staphylococcus aureus* produced 38%, 31.25%, and 19% of the activity of gentamycin against *Staphylococcus aureus* respectively as against the 60%, 55%, and 30% of the anti-*Staphylococcus* activity of gentamycin produced three months earlier by the fresh, ten-year-old, and twenty-year-old lime juice samples. These results suggest that exposure of the lime juice samples to sunlight and air in the laboratory for three months may have lowered the activity of the active ingredients in the lime juice samples that excise activity against Staphylococcus aureus.

The repeat antimicrobial evaluation of fresh lime juice, ten-year-old lime juice, and twenty-year-old lime juice against *Salmonella typhi* produced 65.2%, 70%, and 26% of the anti-*Salmonella-typhi* activity of gentamycin respectively as against the 56%, 60%, and 23% activity they produced three months earlier. These results show that after being on the laboratory shelve for 3 months, fresh, ten-year-old lime juice, and twenty-year-old lime juice samples were even more active against *Salmonella typhi* than were observed when their anti-*Salmonella-typhi* activity was evaluated three months earlier. These results suggest that the activity of the active ingredient of lime juice that acts against Salmonella *typhi* must have increased during the three months' life of the lime juice samples in the laboratory where the antimicrobial evaluations were done. The superiority of the anti-*Salmonella-typhi* activity of ten-year-old lime juice over that of fresh lime juice remained the same for the two evaluations.

The anti-*Bacillus-subtilis* evaluation of fresh lime juice, ten-year-old lime juice, and twenty-year-old lime juice after three months produced 35.2%, 29.4%, and 20.5% of the anti-*Bacillus-subtilis* activity of gentamycin respectively as against the 50%, 45.83%, and 31.32% activity respectively which they produced three months earlier. These results show that handling or exposure of the lime juice samples caused the fresh, ten-year-old lime juice, and twenty-year-old lime juice samples to lose some Bacillus subtilis activity in three months.

The most dramatic result obtained in the repeat evaluation test was the anti-fungal test against *Candida albicans* in which fresh lime juice and ten-year-old and twenty-year-old lime juice samples produced antifungal activity of 171.4%, 171.4%, and 50% the antifungal activity of fluconazole respectively as against the 96%, 92%, and 64% activity they produced three months earlier. Thus the antifungal activity of both the fresh lime juice and ten-year-old lime juice samples were actually 71.4% greater than that of fluconazole, the standard drug, in the repeat antimicrobial evaluation. The antifungal activity of the twenty old lime juice was 50% that of fluconazole in the repeat test. These results suggest that there was a component of lime juice that produces candidacidal activity of lime juice that increased during the three months the fresh and ten-year-old lime juice samples were left on the laboratory shelf where the antimicrobial studies were done.

Conclusions

The results obtained in this evaluation of the antimicrobial activity of fresh, ten-year-old, and twenty-year-old lime juice samples demonstrated the specificity, durability, and longevity of antibacterial and antifungal effects of lime juice. The results obtained demonstrated that lime juice (and by extension, medicinal plant extracts) can produce reproducible beneficial pharmacological effects for the treatment of illnesses, diseases, and health disorders for twenty years or more if properly prepared, packaged, and stored. The results also demonstrated that lime juice (and, by extension, other well prepared and well-stored herbal extracts, juices, or even unextracted medicinal plant materials) can retain valuable activity for many years if properly prepared and stored in dry, cool, dark, clean places and protected from damage.

The antifungal activity of fresh and ten-year-old lime juice samples against *Candida albicans* which increased by 78% and 80% respectively, after being left in the laboratory for three months, suggests that exposure of a medicinal extract or juice to light and or high temperatures can, in some cases, lead to some internal rearrangements in the molecules of their chemical constituents which can increase or decrease some pharmacological activities of the extract or juice.

Below is the report of a comparative preliminary phytochemical screening of the same fresh, ten-year-old, and twenty-year-old lime juice samples which were evaluated for antimicrobial activity.

Preliminary Phytochemical Screening of Fresh, Ten-Year-Stored, and Twenty-Years-Stored Lime Juice to Compare their Composition

1. Utoh-Nedosa Uchechukwu Anastasia

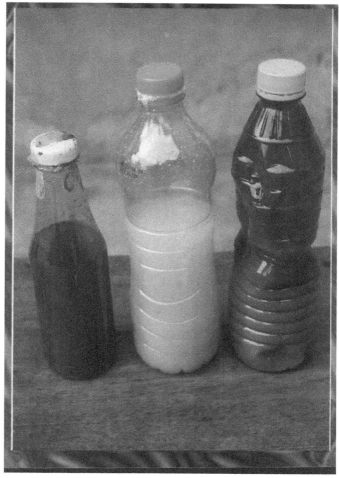

Figure 1. Twenty-year-old lime juice (*left*), fresh lime juice (*middle*), and ten-year-old lime juice (*right*).

Abstract

There has been renewed interest in the plant kingdom both as a source of new drugs and as a source of micronutrients. This study evaluated and compared the phytochemical composition of fresh, ten-year-stored, and twenty-year-stored *Citrus aurantifolia* (Christm. swingle [family Rutaceae]) fruit juice (also called lime juice) to determine its phytochemical composition and pharmacological potentials. Standard phytochemical screening tests were carried out on 5 mL samples of fresh, ten-year-stored, and twenty-year-stored *Citrus aurantifolia* fruit juices. The results of the screening tests showed that each fresh, ten-year-stored, and twenty-year-stored *Citrus aurantifolia* fruit juices contained saponins, tannins, alkaloids, and proteins. Fresh lime juice had the highest saponin and alkaloid content as well as the least tannin content among the three lime juice types. The twenty-year-stored lime juice had the least saponin and alkaloid content as well as the most tannin content, of the three lime juice types. The saponin, alkaloid, and tannin contents of the ten-year-stored lime juice were each midway between that of fresh and twenty-years-stored lime juices. The quantity of the protein content of fresh, ten-year-stored, and twenty-year-stored lime juices was the same. From these results, it is concluded that the quantity of the saponin and alkaloid content of stored lime juice decreases by 1/3 every ten years of storage while the quantity of its tannin content increases by 1/3 every ten years of storage of the lime juice. On the other hand, the protein content of properly stored lime juice remains constant for twenty years. It is also concluded that these findings demonstrate twenty-year durability of pharmacological/medicinal potentials of lime juice which are anchored on its saponin, alkaloid, and tannin contents, and the constancy of its protein content which provide micronutrient and food supplement value.

Keywords: *phytochemical screening, chemical composition, pharmacological potential, fresh, Citrus aurantifolia, lime juice.*

Introduction

As many health disorders and diseases encountered in the late twentieth and early twenty-first century resist total cure and control with orthodox medicines, there has been renewed interest in the plant kingdom both as a source of new drugs and as a source of alternative medicines and micronutrients. Fresh *Citrus aurantifolia* (lime) juice is taken orally in Nigeria as a traditional remedy against gastro-intestinal ailments and disorders. Some users employ lime as a flavoring agent in foods and drinks.[1] Juice of unripe (green) *Citrus aurantifolia* is employed in Nigeria as a powerful scouring or cleaning agent for the removal of thick or greasy dirt, especially from metal containers.

Citrus aurantifolia plants are not abundantly cultivated in Nigeria and the fruit from which lime juice is made is harvested seasonally, necessitating the use of stored lime juice. There is a need therefore to have information on the nature of the constituents of lime juice and how long the active chemical constituents of lime juice remain stable during long periods of storage of lime juice.

Most of the pharmaceutical literature on *Citrus aurantifolia* and other *Citrus* species focus on the oils obtained from their fruit rinds and their leaves.[2], [3], [4] For example, Libyan steam-distilled fresh orange peel was in 1968 found to contain sixty-two components, sixteen of which had never been identified before.[5] Volatile oils, which are known to be present in orange peel, include terpene (+) – limonene, smaller quantities of citral, citronellal, methyl anthranilate, etc.[6]

Since lime juice is part of the lime tree used in Nigerian traditional medicine, this study evaluated and compared the preliminary phytochemical composition of fresh, ten-year-stored, and twenty-year-stored lime juices.

Material and Methods

Citrus aurantifolia (lime) juice was prepared by manual squeezing out of lime juice from the cut surface of the ripe fruit of *Citrus aurantifolia*. The squeezed-out lime juice was then sieved with clean fine-meshed sieves and stored in glass or plastic bottles. The ten-year- and twenty-year-stored lime juice bottles (figure 1, *right* and *left*) were stored in a carton on a bottom shelf in a dimly lit normal room at normal Nigerian room temperature or under a bed in a room lit with a 60 watts electric bulb before bedtime for ten or twenty years. The fresh lime juice (figure 1, *center*), was freshly prepared and used for the study.

The phytochemical composition of fresh, ten-year-stored and twenty-year-stored lime juices was evaluated using standard phytochemical tests described below. The phytochemical composition of freshly prepared lime juice samples was then compared with those of the ten-year-stored and twenty-year-stored lime juice samples.

Phytochemical Screening of the Fresh, Ten-Years-Stored, and Twenty-Year-Stored Lime Juices

The phytochemical analysis of the composition of the fresh, ten-year-stored, and twenty-year-stored lime juices was done by putting 5 mL samples of the fresh, ten-year-stored, and twenty-year-stored lime juices to the following phytochemical screening tests:

Test for Starch

Five mL of fresh, ten-year-stored, and twenty-year-stored lime juice was shaken in 5 mL of distilled water and two drops of iodine were added to it. The nonappearance of blue-black color indicated the absence of starch.

Test for Proteins

Two drops of Millon's reagent were added to 5 mL of fresh, ten-year-stored, and twenty-year-stored lime juice. The appearance of a white precipitate showed the presence of proteins.

Test for Alkaloids

Five mL of fresh, ten-year-stored, and twenty-year-stored lime juice was boiled with 2 mL of dilute HCL in a test tube and filtered. The filtrate was divided into four portions.

Two drops of Meyer's solution were added to portion 1. A white precipitate was obtained, which showed the absence of alkaloids.

Two drops of Wagner's reagent were added to portion 2. A brown precipitate was obtained, which showed the presence of alkaloids.

Two drops of Dragendorff's solution were added to portion 3. An orange precipitate was obtained, which showed the presence of alkaloids.

Two drops of picric acid were added to portion 4. An orange precipitate was obtained, which confirmed the presence of alkaloids in the fresh, ten-year-stored, and twenty-year-stored lime juices.

Test for Flavonoids

Five mL of fresh, ten-year-stored, and twenty-year-stored lime juice was mixed with 5 mL of distilled water in a test tube. Few drops of sodium hydroxide solution were added to the solution. No yellow color was obtained, which showed the absence of flavonoids.

Ten mL of ethyl acetate was added to 5 mL of fresh, ten-year-stored, and twenty-year-stored lime juice and heated on a water bath for three minutes. The mixture was cooled, filtered, and used for the following teats:

a) Ammonium test
   Four mL of the filtrate was shaken with 1 mL of dilute ammonium solution.
   The absence of yellow color in the ammoniacal layer indicated the absence of flavonoids.
b) Ammonium chloride solution (1% test)
   Another 4 mL of the filtrate was shaken with 1 mL of 1% ammonium chloride solution, and the layers were allowed to separate. The absence of yellow color in the ammonium chloride layer indicated the absence of flavonoids.

Test for Tannins

Five mL of fresh, ten-year-stored, and twenty-year-stored lime juice was boiled with 5.0 mL of water filtered and used for the test.

Ferric Chloride Test

Few drops of ferric chloride were added to3ml of the filtrate. A greenish-black precipitate indicated the presence of tannins (elligitannins and gallitannins produced the blue-black color while condensed tannins produced brownish green-brown precipitate).

Test for Saponins

Twenty mL of distilled water was added to 5 mL of fresh, ten-year-stored, and twenty-year-stored lime juice in a test tube and boiled gently in a hot water-bath for twenty minutes. The mixture was filtered hot and allowed to cool. The filtrate was used for the following tests:

a) Frothing test
   Five mL of the filtrate was diluted with 20 mL of distilled water and vigorously shaken and left to stand. A stable foam was observed in the filtrate, which indicated the presence of saponins.
b) Emulsion test
   Two drops of olive oil were added to the frothing solution, and the contents were shaken vigorously. An emulsion was formed from the frothing solution, which showed the presence of saponins.
c) Fehling's test

Five mL of Fehling's solution (equal parts of Fehling's solution A and B) was added to 5 mL of the filtrate, and the content was heated in a water bath. A reddish precipitate, which turned brick red on further heating with added sulfuric acid, indicated the presence of saponins.

Test for Glycosides

Test for Reducing Sugars

Five mL of fresh, ten-year-stored, and twenty-year-stored lime juice was boiled with 10 mL of distilled water. Two mL of Fehling's solution (equal parts of Fehling's solution A and B) was added to the solution, and the contents were heated in a water bath for fifteen minutes. No brick-red precipitate was obtained which showed the absence of reducing sugars.

Sulphuric Acid Test for Glycosides

Three mL of dilute sulphuric acid was added to 5 mL of the resultant solution from test one, and the content was heated for fifteen minutes, cooled, and neutralized with 3 mL potassium hydroxide solution (20%). One mL equal parts mixture of Fehling's solution A and B was added to it and the resultant solution heated for fifteen minutes in a water bath. No brick-red coloration was obtained which showed the absence of glycosides.

Ferric Chloride Test for Glycosides

Three drops of ferric chloride solution were added to another 5 mL of the solution obtained in test one and boiled, cooled, and filtered. The filtrate was shaken with an equal volume of carbon tetrachloride (CCl_4). No lower organic layer separated. Five mL dilute ammonia was added to the test one solution/carbon tetrachloride solution. No red coloration of the solution was obtained, which showed the absence of glycosides.

Ethanol Test and Lead Acetate Test

Twenty mL of 50% ethanol and 10 mL lead acetate solution was added to 5 mL of fresh, ten-year-stored, and twenty-year-stored lime juice and heated in a water bath for 2 minutes, cooled, and filtered. The filtrate was extracted twice with 15 mL aliquots of chloroform. The first chloroform extract was partially evaporated in a water bath and 2 mL aliquots of 3,5-dinitrobenzoic acid solution and 1 mL of sodium hydroxide solution were added to it. No light-violet coloration was observed which showed the absence of glycosides.

The second chloroform extract was evaporated to dryness in a water bath and dissolved in 3 mL glacial acetic acid in a test tube. Two drops of ferric chloride followed by carefully added (by the side of the test tube) 2 mL sulfuric acid was added, and the solution was left to stand for five minutes. No brownish color appeared at the junction of two layers, which confirmed the presence of glycosides in the fresh, ten-year-stored, and twenty-year-stored lime juice.

Results

The phytochemical tests conducted on the fresh, ten-year-stored, and twenty-year-stored *Citrus aurantifolia* fruit juices (lime juice) showed that each of the fresh, ten-year-stored, and twenty-year-stored lime juices contained saponins, tannins, alkaloids, and proteins. The phytochemical tests showed negative results for the presence of flavonoids, glycosides, and carbohydrates in the lime juices.

Fresh lime juice had the highest saponin and alkaloid content as well as the least tannin content among the three lime juice types (table 1). The twenty-year-stored lime juice had the least saponin and alkaloid content as well as the most tannin content of the three lime juice types (table 1). The saponin, alkaloid, and tannin contents of the ten-year-stored lime juice were each midway between that of fresh lime juice and that of twenty-year-old lime juice (table 1). The protein content of fresh, ten-year-stored, and twenty-year-stored lime juices was the same (table 1).

Table 1. The relative chemical composition of fresh, ten-year-stored, and twenty-year-stored lime juices.

	Saponins	Tanins	Flavonoids	Alkaloids	Glycosides	Proteins	Carbohydrates
Lime juice type							
Fresh lime juice	+++	+	−	+++	−	+	−
10 years-stored lime juice	++	++	−	++	−	+	−
20 years-stored lime juice	+	+++	−	+	−	+	−

Discussions

Effect of Storage on Activity of Bioactive Substances

Good storage is aimed at prevention of contamination of a product by extraneous materials and minimization of decomposition of the product, which may arise from chemical, physical and microbiological changes that can occur in a medicinal plant product due to effects of oxygen, humidity/moisture, temperature,[7] and light.[8] The active ingredients of some plant products undergo a rapid change from the presence of enzymes, which are easily activated by moisture[9] or polarized light.[10]

The constituents of some drugs can be deteriorated by oxidation. For example, linseed oil, cannabinol of Indian hemp, oil of turpentine, and oil of lemon are rapidly made resinous by atmospheric oxygen;[11] and cod liver oil thickens, becomes resinous, and darkens in color with long exposure to air.[12]

The results of this study showed that the proportion of the initial active ingredients of lime juice decreased or increased with time. The quantity of the saponins and alkaloids in the lime juice gradually reduced by a third every ten years while the quantity of the tannin content of the lime juice increased by a third every ten years to produce the greenish-brown ten-year-old lime juice and the reddish-brown twenty-year-old lime juice seen in figure 1. It is possible that there was a chemical conversion of the saponins and or alkaloids to tannins as the lime juice passed from fresh to twenty-year-old lime juice. However, the interesting thing is that lime juice continued to demonstrate pharmacological and medicinal properties with time, which shows that the medicinal effects of lime juice reside in its saponins, alkaloids, and tannins with the support of its protein contents.

The study concludes that the quantity of the saponin and alkaloid content of lime juice decreases by 1/3 every ten years of storage while the quantity of its tannin content increases by 1/3 every ten years of storage of the lime juice and the quantity of its protein content remains constant for twenty years. It is also concluded that the pharmacological and medicinal effects of lime juice are anchored on its saponin, alkaloid, and tannin contents supported by its protein content. Since the saponin-, alkaloid- and tannin- contents of the twenty-year-old lime juice were still fairly high when they were evaluated, it is possible that the twenty-year-old lime juice could demonstrate pharmacological and medicinal activity for another five or more years. Further studies will verify that.

References

1. Y. A. Ramesh et al., "Flavour Quality of Dehydrated lime (Citrus aurantifolia [Christm. Swindle])," Food Chemistry 85, 1 (2004): 59–61.
2. O. Ekundayo et al., "The Composition of Petitgrain Oil (Citrus limon), N. L. Burm," Journal of Essential Oil Research 2 (1990): 269–270.
3. O. Ekundayo et al., "Nigeria Sweet Orange Leaf Oil Composition," Journal of Essential Oil Research 2 (1990): 329–330.
4. O. Ekundayo et al., "Leaf Volatile Oil Composition of Mandarin (Citrus reticulate)," Journal of Essential Oil Research 2 (1990): 199–201.
5. O. Ekundayo et al., "The Composition of Petitgrain Oil (Citrus limon), N. L. Burm," Journal of Essential Oil Research 2 (1990): 269–270.
6. Ibid.
7. G. Trueman, "Effect of Temperature on Intravenous Solutions and Peritoneal Dialysis Fluids after Shelf Storage and Incubation in Climatic Cabinet," Journal of Hospital Pharmacy 31: 239–242.
8. William Charles Evans, Trease and Evans Pharmacognosy, 16th ed. (Edinburgh: Saunders Elsevier, 2009).
9. Ibid.
10. J. R. Walmsley, "Everyday Problems in the Pharmacy," Pharmacy Journal (1930): 125–507.
11. William Charles Evans, Trease and Evans Pharmacognosy, 16th ed. (Edinburgh: Saunders Elsevier, 2009).
12. Ibid.

CHAPTER 12

Commonalities in the Effects of Extracts and Juices of Medicinal Plants on the Body of their Recipients

WHEN A MEDICINAL plant extract or juice is taken into the body of an organism, it gets absorbed into the tissues of the organism through tiny pores on the surface of cells called cell surface receptors. Once inside the cells of the host, medicinal plant extracts elicit or produce some effects in the organism for some time at the end of which the extract gets broken down or metabolized by the body of the organism to produce some byproducts of the extract (or constituent of the extract). The byproducts or metabolites of the plant extract are finally removed from the body through the excretory processes of the organism. This chapter links the effects of medicinal plant extracts and juices felt at the tissues and organs of the body where they are produced to the mechanism by which these effects are produced in the body of organisms.

The effects of plants of four medicinal plant families will be used to show the mechanisms by which medicinal plants interact with the body of organisms.

The four plant families are family *Leguminosae*, family *Annonaceae*, family *Caricaceae*, family *Anacardiaceae*, and family *Cucurbitaceae*.

The effects of the plant extracts (and/or their constituents) described in the scientific researches documented on plants of family *Leguminosae*, family *Annonaceae*, family *Caricaceae*, and family *Cucurbitaceae* will be summarized below to identify the common denominator in the effects.

Table 1. A summary of the medicinal effects of plants of family Leguminosaceae, which were described in chapter 5, to indicate the nature of these effects on the body of the host organism.

Plant	Its Activity or Effect	Nature of This Activity
Indigofera arrecta	Antidiabetic activity	Inhibition of hyperglycemia
Indigofera arrecta	Anti-ulcerogenic activity	Inhibition of ulcer
Pilostigma thonningii	Antibacterial activity	Inhibition or killing of bacteria

(c-methylflavonoids)	Inhibition of prostaglandin synthesis	Inhibition
Tetrapleura tetraptera		
Methyl extract of *Tetrapleura tetraptera*	Inhibition and killing of *Bulinus globosus*	Inhibition
Water extract of *Tetrapleura tetraptera*	Inhibition and killing of *Biomphalaria galabrata*	Inhibition
	Slowing of the heart of *Biophalaria galabrata*	Inhibition
Volatile oils from fresh fruits of *Tetrapleura tetraptera*	Protection of mice from leptazol-induced convulsions	Inhibition of convulsion
Scopoletin isolated from powdered *Tetrapleura tetraptera*	Hypotensive effects: inhibition of contractions of the artery, attenuation of contraction of rabbit duodenum, depression of contraction of chick esophagus	Inhibition of contraction Inhibition of contraction Inhibition of contraction
Aridan isolated from *Tetrapleura tetraptera*	Reduction of egg production of *Biomphalaria galabrata* snails	Inhibition of egg production
	Produced significant reductions of glycogen of *Biomphalaria galabrata*	Inhibition of glycogen builds up
Ciliandra portoricensis (aqueous root and stem extract)	Anticonvulsant activity in mice	Inhibition of convulsion
Ciliandra portoricensis (root extract)	Sustained contraction of guinea pig ileum blocked by atropine	Production of contraction
Daniella oliveri (ethanol extract)	Antimicrobial activity	Inhibition of microbial growth
	Inhibition of histamine-induced contraction of guinea pig ileum and Ach-induced contraction of frog rectus abdominis muscle	Inhibition of contraction Inhibition of contraction
Daniella oliveri (Hexane extract)	Analgesic activity	Inhibition of pain
Daniella oliveri (Methanol extract)	Anti-inflammatory activity Inhibition of contraction	Inhibition of inflammation
Baphia nitida (leaf extract)	Anti-inflammatory activity	Inhibition of inflammation
Detarium microcarpum (stem bark extract)	Analgesic and anti-inflammatory activity	Inhibition of pain and Inhibition of inflammation
Mucuna prurens	Antimicrobial activity	Inhibition of microbial growth

Dialium guineense (fruit and leaf extract)	Moluscicidal activity	The killing of parasites harbored by mollusks (snails) (inhibition of parasitic infection)
Parkia biglobosa and *Parkia bicolor*	Antibacterial and antifungal activity	The killing of fungi and inhibition of fungal growth
Cassia occidentalis	Laxative activity	Gentle contraction of intestinal walls to move feces for expulsion
	Antimalarial activity	The killing of malarial parasites and Inhibition of escalation of malaria
	Toxic cardiomyopathy	(Excessive depressive contraction of the myocardium leading to damage of heart muscles)
	Protection against chromosomal aberrations	Inhibition of chromosomal damage
Cassia podocarpa	Laxative and purgative activity,	Gentle and strong contractions of intestinal muscles to produce laxative and purgative activity.

Table 2. A summary of the medicinal effects of plants of family Anonnaceae, which were described in chapter 4, to indicate the nature of these effects on the body of the host organism.

Plant	Its Activity or Effect	Nature of This Activity
Enantia chlorantha	Anti-malarial activity	The killing of malarial parasites and Inhibition of escalation of malaria
Aqueous of *Enantia chlorantha*	Antipyretic activity in rabbits	Inhibition of fever
Aqueous extract of *Enantia chlorantha*	Analgesic activity in rabbits	Inhibition of pain
Volatile oil of *Dennettia tripetalla* seed	Antifungal activity	The killing of fungi and inhibition of fungal growth
Aqueous extract of *Xylopia aethiopica* seed	Lowered intraocular pressure	Inhibition of excessive increases in intra-ocular pressure

Aqueous extract of *Xylopia aethiopica* seed	Reduced near point of (visual) convergence	Inhibition of increase in near point of convergence of visual light
Aqueous extract of *Xylopia aethiopica* seed	Inhibition to increase amplitude of accommodation	Excitation to increase the amplitude of accommodation
Essential oils of *Xylopia aethiopica* fruit	Antibacterial activity	The killing of bacteria and inhibition of bacterial growth
Essential oils of *Xylopia aethiopica* fruit	Antifungal activity	Promoted dislodging, granulation and healing, and reduced odor in chronic ulcers
Essential oils of *Monodora myristica*	Antibacterial activity	The killing of bacteria and inhibition of bacterial growth
Essential oils of *Monodora myristica* fruits	Antifungal activity	The killing of fungi and inhibition of fungal growth
Aqueous and methanol extract of *Xylopia aethiopica* fruit	Inhibited intestinal propulsive movements in rats	Inhibition of intestinal propulsive movements in rats
Essential oils of *Xylopia aethiopica* fruit	Showed cytotoxic activity to cancer cells	The killing of cancer cells and inhibition of growth of cancer cell lines
Kaurene derivative of *Xylopia aethiopica* fruit extract	Produced cardiotonic, diuretic, and natriuretic activity similar to those of chlorothiazide	Gentle stimulation of cardiac muscles and promotion of diuresis and natriuresis

Table 3. A summary of the medicinal effects of plants of family *Caricaceae*, which were described in chapter 6, to indicate the nature of these effects on the body of the host organism.

Plant	Its Activity or Effect	Nature of this Activity
Extract of mature unripe *Carica papaya* (pawpaw) fruit	Anti-diabetic activity comparable to Chlorpropamide	Inhibition of hyperglycemia
Milled *Carica papaya* seed	Antinematodiasis (helminth infection), activity in village goats	Inhibition of helminthic infection
Carica papaya seed extract	Inhibited apoptosis in cultured U937 cells in human monocyte/ macrophage cell line	Inhibition of macrophages Anticancer effects
Carica papaya unripe fruit juice	Antihypertensive effect in renal and DOCA-induced hypertension in rats	Inhibition of hypertension

The derivative of papain (juice of unripe pawpaw fruit), chymopapain	Dissolves the nucleus of the intervertebral disc in cases of herniated lumber or trapped nerves in orthopedic surgery	Inhibition of blockage of intervertebral disc joints.
Chloroform extract of *Carica papaya* seeds	Decreased the sperm concentration in langur monkeys	Excessive inhibitory activity leading to inhibition spermatogenesis
Chloroform extract of *Carica papaya* seeds	Exhibited abortifacient properties on female Sprague-Dawley rats	Excessive inhibitory activity leading to inhibition of fetal anchorage and development
Extract of dried fruits of *Carica papaya*	Exhibited protective effects on hepatotoxicity	Inhibition of liver toxicity and liver damage
Topical application of the juice of unripe fruit of pawpaw	Promoted dislodging, granulation and healing, and reduced odor in chronic ulcers	Inhibition of exasperation and expansion of ulcer by promoting expired cell dislodging, wound granulation and healing, and reduced odor in chronic ulcers
Topical application of the juice of unripe fruit of pawpaw	Were effective in dislodging necrotic tissue and preventing infection of burns	Inhibition of infection of burns and inhibition of prolongation of stay of necrotic tissue
The latex or sap of *Carica papaya*	Exhibited antifungal properties	Killing of fungi and inhibition of fungal growth
The latex or sap of *Carica papaya*	Exhibited anti-amoeba properties	Killing of amoeba and inhibition of amoebic growth amoebic infections
The latex of the unripe fruit of pawpaw and crystalline papain	Produced anti-ulcer effects by significantly reducing histamine-induced acid secretion in chronic gastric fistulated-rats	Inhibition of histamine-induced acid secretion in chronic gastric fistulated-rats, thereby inhibiting the progression of the ulcers
Extract of unripe papaya	Antibacterial activities	The killing of bacteria and inhibition of bacterial growth
Extract of unripe papaya	Antioxidant activities comparable to those of soybean paste miso, rice bran, and baker's yeast.	Inhibition of damaging oxidative activities of reactive oxygen species and oxidative stress from other sources
Seed and pulp of *Carica papaya*	Antioxidant activities comparable to those of soybean paste miso; rice bran and baker's yeast	Inhibition of oxidative stress

Table 4. A summary of the medicinal effects of plants of the family *Cucurbitaceae*, which were described in chapter 6, to indicate the nature of these effects on the body of the host organism.

Plant	Its Activity or Effect	Nature of This Activity
In vivo administration of *Momordica charantia* extracts in Sprague-Dawley rats	Caused a decrease in muscle and liver glycogen	Inhibition of increases in muscle and liver glycogen
in vivo administration of *Momordica charantia* extracts in Sprague-Dawley rats	Caused an increase in muscle and liver protein levels	Inhibition of protein breakdown in liver and muscle, and stimulation of Protein *synthesis*.
In vivo administration of *Momordica charantia* extracts in Sprague-Dawley rats	Produced decrease in brain protein	Stimulation of protein utilization in the brain
In vivo administration of *Momordica charantia* extracts in Sprague-Dawley rats	Caused a decrease in the activities of serum L-alanine transaminase and alkaline phosphatase	Inhibition of the activities of serum l-alanine transaminase enzyme.
In vivo administration of *Momordica charantia* extracts in Sprague-Dawley rats	Caused a decrease in the activities of alkaline phosphatase	Inhibition of the activities of alkaline phosphatase enzyme
The ethanol extract of *Momordica charantia*	Did not affect the level of the activity of L-aspartate transaminase	Elicitation of both inhibition and excitation (biphasic effect), resulting in not affecting the level of the activity of L-aspartate transaminase
The ethanol extract of *Momordica charantia*	Decreased the activity of adenosine triphosphatase	Inhibition of the activity of adenosine triphosphatase (which amounts to lowering the energy in the medium) to basal levels
Momordica charantia extract	Significantly ($P < 0.05$) reduced the fasting blood sugar levels of both normal and diabetic rats by 37.69% and 145.8% respectively	Inhibition of hyperglycaemia. Anti-diabetic activity.
Momordica charantia extract	Increased the activity of erythrocyte Ca^{2+} ATPase in the alloxan-induced diabetic rabbits by 67.57% but not in controls	Inhibition of ATP. Inhibition of excessive energy utilization by body cells.

Momordica charantia extract	Slightly raised the activity of the calcium pump of the intestinal mucosa of the extract-treated alloxan-induced diabetic rabbits in comparison with those of controls.	Inhibition of hyperglycemia by low energy stimulation of glucose utilization by intestinal mucosa of diabetic rabbits
"Charantin" isolates from *Mormodica charantia* seed extract	Was found to be more potent than tolbutamide in hypoglycaemic activity	Potent inhibition of hyperglycaemia. Potent anti-diabetic effects.
Foetidin was isolated from *Momordica foetida* seed extract	Was found to be more potent than tolbutamide in hypoglycaemic activity	Potent inhibition of hyperglycaemia and Potent anti-diabetic effects.
Extracts of the roots of *Momordica augustisepala*[27]	Exhibited abortifacient effects	Excessive inhibition activity resulting in exhibition of abortifacient effects
Extract of the fruit of *Lagenaria breviflora*	Anti-implantation activity	Uterine contraction activity resulting in oxytocin-like or oxytocic activity.
Extract of the fruit of *Lagenaria breviflora*	Exhibited oxytocic activity	Excitation activity resulting in anti-oxytocic activity

Discussions of Results

The type of effects plants of family *Leguminosae* produced in the body add up to twenty-eight inhibitory responses and two excitatory responses (figure 1). This suggests that twenty-six out of twenty-eight effects of plants of the *Leguminosae* family (beans and peas) would be inhibitory effects in the body while the remaining two would be excitatory effects. One of the few excitatory effects they produce is a laxative effect. Thus, when consumed as food or when taken as medicine, pharmacologically active constituents of their extracts produce largely inhibitory responses in the body which relax or calm agitated organs or tissues of the body. Occasionally, like when taken in excessive amounts (or when taken in normal amounts by a few individuals who are slow metabolizers of their active ingredients, and sometimes also slow metabolizers of many other substances), products of plants of family *Leguminosae* will produce excitatory effects. Among the papers cited in the references below, thirty-eight papers[2–20, 21–27, 28–39] reported inhibitory effects of plants of family *Leguminosae* while only four papers[40, 41, 42, 43] reported excitatory effects of plants of family *Leguminosae*.

The types of effects plants of family *Annonaceae* produce in the body tabulated in figure 2 add up to fifteen inhibitory responses and one excitatory response. Thus, fifteen out of sixteen effects of plants of the family *Annonaceae* were inhibitory or relaxation responses in the body. This means that juices and extracts of plants of family *Annonaceae* like soursop and Ethiopian pepper, produce mainly inhibitory effects. One out of sixteen of reported effects of plants of family *Annonaceae* producing an occasional excitatory response as is largely done by some members of plants of family *Annonaceae* like *Xylopia aethiopica* and *Dennetia tripetella*, which contain some acidic compounds like *Xylopia aethiopica* that contains xylopic acid. This position is substantiated by the effects of plants of family *Annonaceae* cited in the references below in which fourteen articles reported inhibitory effects of plants of family *Annonaceae*[44–58] and only one article reported the elicitation of an excitatory response by a plant of this family.[59]

A summary of the excitatory and inhibitory pharmacological effects of plants of family *Caricaceae* in the body, tabulated in figure 3, shows that they add up to seventeen inhibitory responses and zero excitatory response.[10][60–76] Thus, if one administered extracts of leaves, fruits, stem barks, or seeds of plants of family *Caricaceae* for the correction of any health disorders in humans, plants, or animals, all extracts without exception would exhibit inhibitory or relaxation response in the body. Relaxation or inhibitory response antagonize or inhibit any stressful or excitatory condition in the body in which the inhibitory responses produced. This also means that juices and extracts of plants of family *Caricaceae* like pawpaw plant (whether used alone or in combination with another medicinal substance) will always make an inhibitory input.

In the case of plants of the family *Cucurbitaceae* listed in table 4, their inhibitory and excitatory effects add up to sixteen inhibitory responses and two excitatory responses. This shows that extracts of plants of family *Cucurbitaceae* (which include pumpkins, squashes, cucumber and melon species) produce mostly inhibitory effects in the body like plants of family *Caricaceae*, but the constituents of a few of the members of the family like *Mormordica charantia* can in some occasions produce excitatory effects.[77, 78, 79]

Conclusion

Out of eighty-three research articles reviewed here for the medicinal effects of plants of family *Leguminosae*, family *Annonaceae*, family *Caricaceae*, and family *Cucurbitaceae*, seventy-seven of them exhibited inhibitory pharmacological effects (which is also equivalent to inhibitory physiological activity effects) while only six articles reported excitatory activity of the extracts. This is equivalent to saying that 93% of the pharmacological and physiological actions of medicinal plant extracts are inhibitory while 7% of the pharmacological and physiological actions of medicinal plant extracts are excitatory. This is in line with the role of remediation of disordered conditions of the body of humans, animals, or other plants which medicinal plant extracts are called upon to play when the body is disordered or damaged by disease or destructive biochemical, chemical, or other agents. When the body is functioning normally, medicinal plant extracts have only a disease or health disorder preventive role to play, which is also a health disorder-inhibitory role.

The 7% excitatory effects exhibited by plant extracts encountered in this review suggest that plant extracts only exhibit occasional excitatory roles when that excitation is a necessary component of the disease and health disorder preventive or curative role of the plant extracts. For example, *Cassia occidentalis* produced antimalarial activity, protection from chromosomal aberrations, and laxative activity. It was probably taken in a fairly high dose to relieve constipation, for it to produce the laxative activity. *Cassia podocarpa*, which is another species of cassia, on the other hand, produced both laxative and purgative activity. These two different speeds of stool evacuation effects of *Cassia podocarpa* suggest that the medicinal component that produced the intestinal or colon smooth muscle contractions that produce the laxative or purgative effects respectively (which is likely to be the anthraquinone component) is present in larger amounts in extracts of *Cassia podocarpa* than they are in extracts of *Cassia occidentalis*.

Again, some medicinally active constituents of plant extracts and juices may excise excitatory activity in body tissues or glands of the host body to stimulate the secretion of substances needed to enhance the performance of the body like stimulation of the production of hormones, mucus, saliva, tear et cetera. An example of such excise of excitatory action is the baby at-term-ejection role of castor oil when it is used medically in obstetrics for the induction of labor in hypertensive patients whose labor must be induced to deliver the baby before the pregnant woman goes into normal labor to prevent her going into hypertensive crisis while laboring. In this fetus-ejection action, castor oil exercises an oxytocin-like contraction action on uterine smooth muscles to eject the baby whose delivery is induced. Another two examples are the cough expectorant effect of *Annona muricata*, soursop fruit pulp, and the cough suppressive effect of *Garcinia kola* seed extract in which the soursop pulp or juice and the *Garcina kola* seed extract directly inhibit respiratory tract smooth muscles to produce their effects.

In conclusion, the nature of the effects of medicinal plant extracts and juices observed in much scientific research, including those cited in this chapter and other chapters of this book, is that most plant extracts and juices produce predominantly inhibitory effects and occasional excitatory effects in the body of their host organisms; and this is what enables them to play disease and body disorder preventive and corrective roles in the body.

References

1. A. K Nyarko, A. A. Sittie, and M. E. Addy, "The basis for the anti-glycaemic activity of Indigofera arrecta in the rat," Phytother Res. 7 (1993): 1–4.
2. A. A. Sittie and A. K. Nyako, "Indigofera arrecta: safety evaluation of an anti-diabetic plant extract in nondiabetic human volunteers," Phytother Res. 12, 1 (1998): 52–54.
3. "Anti-ulcerogenic activity of hot aqueous extract of powdered Indigofera affecta, in vivo," Wambebe (2000), www.sciweb.com/features/patents/patents.
4. J. C. Ibewuike et al., "Anti-inflammatory and anti-bacterial activities of C-methylflavonoids from Piliostigma thonningii (1997).
5. J. A. Ojewale and S. K. Adesina, "Mechanism of the hypotensive effect of Scopoletin isolated from the fruit of Tetrapleura tetraptera," Planta. Medica 49 (1983): 46–50.
6. C. O. Adewunmi, "Water extract of Tetrapleura tetraptera: an effective molluscicide for the control of Schistosomiasis and Fascioliasis in Nigeria," Journal of Animal Production and Research 4, 1 (1984): 73–84.
7. J. I. Nwaiwu and P. A. Akah, "Anticonvulsant effect of the volatile oil from the fruit of Tetrapleura tetraptera," Journal of Ethnopharmacology 18, 2 (1986): 103–107.
8. P. A. Akah and J. I. Nwaiwu, "Anticonvulsant activity of root and stem extracts of Calliandra portoricensis," Journal of Ethnopharmacology 22, 2 (1988): 205–210.
9. C. O. Adewunmi, P. Furu, and H. Madsen, "Evaluation of the effects of low concentrations of Aridanin isolated from Tetrapleura tetraptera Taub. (Mimosaceae), on the growth and egg production of Biomphalaria glabrata and Lymanaea columella Say," Phytotherapy Research 3, 3 (1989): 81–84.
10. C. O. Adewunmi, W. Becker, and G. Dorfler, "Effect of prolonged administration of sublethal concentration of Aridanin isolated from Tetrapleura tetraptera and Bayluscide on the glycogen and protein content of Biomphalaria glabrata," Journal of Ethnopharmacology 24 (1988): 107–114.
11. C. O. Adewunmi, G. Dorfler, and W. Becker, "Effect of Aridanin isolated from Tetrapleura tetraptera and serotonin on the isolated gastrointestinal tract smooth muscle of Biomphalaria glabrata and uptake of calcium," Journal of Natural Products 53 (1990): 956–959.
12. S. Ntiejumokwu and D. N. Onwukaeme, "Antimicrobial and Preliminary Phytochemical Screening of the Leaves of Daniella oliveri (Rolfe) Hutch and Dalz (Leguminosae)," West African Journal of Pharmacology and Drug Research 9, 10 (1991): 95–99.
13. N. D. Onwukaeme, "Anti-inflammatory activities of flavonoids of Baphia nitida Lodd. (Leguminosae), on mice and rats," Journal of Ethnopharmacology 46, 2 (1995): 121–124.
14. J. C. Aguiyi et al., "Antimicrobial activity and preliminary phytochemical screening of the seed of Mucuna pruriens, (Linn) DC," West African Journal of Biological Sciences 5, 1 (1996): 71–76.

15. A. U. D. Bode et al., "The effects of extracts from Tetrapleura tetraptera (Taub.) and Bayluscide on cells and tissue structures of Biomphalaria glabrata (Say.)," Journal of Ethnopharmacology 50 (1996): 103–113.

16. R. Nia et al., "Adesina Antibacterial Constituents of Calliandra haematocepala," Nigerian Journal of Natural Products and Medicine 3 (1999): 58–60.

17. E. Ajaiyeoba, "Phytochemical and anti-bacterial properties of Parkia biglobosa and Parkia bicolor (Mimosaceae) leaf extracts," African Journal of Biomedical Research 5 (2002): 125–129.

18. L. Tona et al., "In vivo antimalarial activity of Cassia occidentalis, Morinda morindoides and Phyllantus niruri," Drug Chem. Toxicol. 20, 2 (1999): 643–53.

19. N. Sharma et al., "Protective effect of Cassia occidentalis extract on chemical-induced chromosomal aberrations in mice," Ann. Trop. Med. And Parasitol. 95, 1 (2001): 47–57.

20. P. J. O'Hara and K. R. Pierce, "Toxic cardiomyopathy caused by Cassia occidentalis, 11 Biochemical studies in poisoned rabbits," Vet. Pathol. 11 (1974): 110–124.

21. S. Damodaran and S. Venkataraman, "A study on the therapeutic efficacy of Cassia alata leaf extract against Pityriasis versicolor," J. Ethnopharmacol 42, 1 (1994): 19–23.

22. S. Palanichamy and S. J. Nagarajan, "Analgesic activity of Cassia alata leaf extract and kaempferol-3-O-sophoroside," Ethnopharmacol 29, 1 (1990): 73–78.

23. E. O. Iwalewa et al., "In vitro anti-malarial activity of leaf extracts of Cassia occidentalis and Guiera senegalensis on Plassmodium yoelii nigerensis," West African Journal of Pharmacology and Drug Research 4 (1990): 19–21.

24. J. A. Onaolapo, P. P. Rai, and E. N. Sokomba, "Preliminary study on the antimicrobial activities of Cassia tora and Cassia occidentalis," Glimpsies in Plant Research 11 (1993): 533–536.

25. E. O. Iwalewa et al., "In vivo and In vitro anti-malarial activity of two leaf extracts of Cassia occidentalis leaf," Nigerian Journal of Pharmaceutical Sciences 5 (1997): 23–28.

26. B. E. Akinde, I. Okeke, and O.O. Orafidiya, "Phytochemical and anti-bacterial evaluations of Cassia alata leaf extract," West African Journal of Pharmacy 13, 1 (1999): 36–40.

27. A. A. Elujoba, A. T. Abere, and S. A. Adelusi, "Laxative properties of Cassia pods sourced from Nigeria," Nigerian Journal of Natural Products and Medicine 3 (1999): 51–53.

28. A. A. Adekunle, "Antifungal property of the crude extract of Brachystegia eurycoma and Richardia brasilensis," Nigerian Journal of Natural Products and Medicine 4 (2000): 70–72.

29. F. C. Chidume et al., "Anti-nociceptive and smooth muscle contracting activities of methanol extract of Cassia tora leaf," Journal of Ethnopharmacology 81, 2 (2002): 205-209.

30. B. E. Akinde, O. O. Oradifaya, and A. O. Oyedele, "The effect of time of collection and storage on the antifungal activity of fresh Cassia alata Linn (Caesalpinaceae) aqueous leaf extract from old and young leaves," Nigerian Journal of Pharmaceutical Research 1, 1 (2002): 95–96.

31. O. Obiageri et al., "Antimicrobial screening of extracts and fractions of Cassia nigrans Vahl (Caesalpinacea) and their effects on Helicobacter pylori," Nigerian Journal of Natural Products and Medicine 7 (2003): 82.

32. C. F. Anowi et al., "Evaluation of antidiarrhoeal activity of the methanolic/methylene (50:50) of the leaves of Desmodium velitinum Fam Fabaceae," IJPI's Journal of Pharmacognosy and Herbal Formulations, www.ijpijournals.com.

33. Anowi Chinedu Fred et al., "Antipyretic and phytochemical evaluation of the ethanol extract of the leaves of Desmodium velutinum," Asian Journal of Pharmacy and Life Sciences 2, 2 (2012): 340–345.

34. Anowi Chinedu Fred et al., "An investigation into the antipyretic activity of n-hexane extract of the leaves of Baphia pubescens. Hook F. Family Leguminosae," JPP (Journal of Pharmacognosy and Phytochemistry) 3, 2 (2014): 127–131.

35. Anowi Chinedu Fredrick et al., "Anti-inflammatory, phytochemical and toxicological investigations of ethanol extract of the leaves of Baphia pubescens Hook F (family Leguminosae)," AJBPR (Asian Journal of Biochemical and Pharmaceutical Research) 2, 4 (2014).

36. Anowi Chinedu Fredrick et al., "An investigation into the anti-inflammatory activity of n-hexane extract of the leaves of Baphia pubescens Hook F (family Leguminosae)," JPCBS (Journal of Pharmaceutical, Chemical and Biological Sciences) 2, 2 (2014).

37. Anowi Chinedu Fredrick et al., "Analgesic, phyochemical and toxicological investigations of ethanol extract of the leaves of Baphia pubescens Hook, Family Leguminosae," Universal Journal of Pharmacy 3, 4 (2014): 11–16.

38. Anowi Chinedu Fredrick et al., "Antipyretic, phytochemical and toxicological investigations of ethanol extract of the leaves of Baphia pubescens Hook. F (Family: Leguminosae)," IJPPR (International Journal of Pharmaceutical and Phytopharmacological Research) 5, 2 (2015): 1–8.

39. Uchechukwu Anastasia Utoh-Nedosa et al., "The Mechanism of Medicinal Effects of Soursop (Annona muricata) Plant Extracts," Inventi Rapid: Ethnopharmacology 2011, no. 3 (September 2011).

40. S. Palanichamy, "Antifungal activity of Cassia alata leaf extract," J. Ethnopharmacol 29, 3 (1990): 337–340.

41. K. A. Abo, S. W. Lasaki, and A. A. Adeyemi, "Laxative and anti-microbial properties of Cassia species growing in Ibadan," Nigerian Journal of Natural Products and Medicine 3 (1999): 47–50.

42. A. A. Adekunle, "Antifungal property of the crude extract of Brachystegia eurycoma and Richardia brasilensis," Nigerian Journal of Natural Products and Medicine 4 (2000): 70–72.

43. B. E. Akinde, O. O. Oradifaya, and A. O. Oyedele, "The effect of time of collection and storage on the antifungal activity of fresh Cassia alata Linn (Caesalpinaceae) aqueous leaf extract from old and young leaves," Nigerian Journal of Pharmaceutical Research 1, 1 (2002): 95–96.

44. Uchechukwu Anastasia Utoh-Nedosa et al., "The Mechanism of Medicinal Effects of Soursop (Annona muricata) Plant Extracts," Inventi Rapid: Ethnopharmacology 2011, no. 3 (September 2011).

45. A. C. Kudi et al., "Screening of some Nigerian medicinal plants for anti-bacterial activity," Journal of Ethnopharmacology 67, 2 (1999): 225–228.

46. J. A. O. Ojewole, "Hypoglycemic effect of Sclerocarya birrea {(A. Rich) Hochst} (Anacardiaceae) Stem-bark Aqueous Extract in Rats," Phytomedicine 10 (2003): 675–681.

47. "Evaluation of the anti-inflammatory properties of Sclerocarya birrea {(A. Rich) Hochst} (family: Anacardiaceae) Stem-bark Extracts in Rats," Journal of Ethnopharmacology 85, 2–3 (2003): 217–220.

48. L. I. Somova et al., "Cardiovascular and diuretic activity of kaurene derivatives of Xylopia aethiopica and Alepidea amatymbica," J. Ethnopharmacol 77, 2–3 (2001): 165–74.

49. S. A. Igwe, J. C. Afonne, and S. I. Ghasic, "Ocular dynamics of systemic aqueous extracts of Xylopia aethiopica (African guinea pepper) seeds on visually active volunteers," J. of Ethnopharmacol 86, 2–3 (2003): 139–142.

50. O. O. Ebong, B. A. Wariso, and I. Orupabo, "The gastrointestinal inhibitory actions of Xylopia aethiopicum (Dunal) A Rich (Annonaceae) in rats," West African Journal of Pharmacology and Drug Research 11 (1995): 94–98.

51. O. T. Asekun and B. A. Adeniyi, "Antimicrobial and cytotoxic activities of the fruit essential oil of Xylopia aethiopica from Nigeria," Fitoterapia 75, 3–4 (2004): 386–370.

52. K. Boakye-Yiadom, N. Fiagbe, and S. Ayim, "Antimicrobial properties of some West African medicinal plants IV. Antimicrobial activity of Xylopic acid and other constituents of the fruits of Xylopia aethiopica (Annonaceae)," Lloydia 40, 6 (1977): 543–545.

53. L. N. Tatsadjieu et al., "Antibacterial and antifungal activity of Xylopia aethiopica, Monodora mystica, Zanthoxylum xanthoxyloides and Zanthoxylum leprieuril from Cameroon," Fitoterapia 74, 5 (2003): 469–472.

54. N. R. Isu, "A survey of the antibacterial effect of some edible spices: Afromomum meleguata, Xylopia aethiopica and Ocimum viride," Nigerian Journal of Natural Products and Medicine 7 (2003): 69.

55. U. A. Utoh-Nedosa, "Evaluation of the Antimicrobial Effects of Ethanol and Water Extract of Dry Fruits of Xylopia aethiopica (Duna) A. Rich on bacterial and fungal isolates," International Conference on Traditional Medicine, Jos (February 21–26, 2016).

56. E. O. Agbaje and A. O. Onabanjo, "Analgesic and Antipyretic Actions of Anantia chloratha extract in some laboratory animals," Nigerian Journal of Natural Products and Medicine (1998): 2.

57. E. O. Ajaiyeoba et al., "Synthesis and antifungal activities of 2-phenylnitroethane; a component of Dennettia tripetalla fruits and Nitro vinyl Derivatives," Journal of Pharmaceutical Research and Development 4, 1 (1999): 47–52.

58. Chrissie S. Abaidoo, Eric Woode, and Abass Alhassan, "An evaluation of the effect of ethanolic fruit extracts of Xylopia aethiopica on haematological and biochemical parameters in male rats," Der Pharmacia Sinca 2, 2 (2011): 39–45.

59. Eze Kingsley Nwangwa, "Anti-fertility effects of ethanolic extract of Xylopia aethiopica on male reproductive organ of Wistar rats," American Journal of Medicine and Medical Sciences 2, 1 (2012): 12–15.

60. J. M. Oke, "Anti-diabetic potency of pawpaw, Carica papaya," African Journal of Biomedical Research 1 (1998): 31–34.

61. M. A. Dipeolu, D. Eruvbetine, and M.O. Abiola, "Potentials of pawpaw (Carica papaya seeds as treatment for nematodiasis in village goats)," Bioprospector 1, 1 (1999): 15–20.

62. O. Dosumu et al., "Carica papaya extract enhances cellular response to stress in U937," Nigerian Journal of Health and Biomedical Sciences 2, 2 (2003): 94–97.

63. A. E. Eno et al., "Blood pressure depression by the fruit juice of Carica papaya (L) in renal and DOCA-induced hypertension in rats," Phytotherapy Res. 14, 4 (2000): 235–239.

64. Purdue University, "Papaya: Carica papaya L.," http://www.hort.purdue.edu/newcrop/morton/papaya ars.html.

65. G. D. Pamplona-Roger, "Papaya Tree-Digestive and Vermifuge," in Encyclopaedia of Medicinal Plants: Education and Health Library (Toledo, Spain: Artes Graficas, 1998), 1435.

66. N. K. Lohiya et al., "Chloroform extract of Carica papaya induces long-term reversible azoospermia in langur monkey," Asian J Androl 4 (2002): 17–26.

67. O. Oderinde et al., "Abortifacient properties of aqueous extract of Carica papaya (linn) seeds on female Sprague-Dawley rats," Nier Postgraduate Med. J. 9, 2 (2002): 95–98.

68. B. Rajikapoor et al., "Effect of dried fruits of Carica papaya on hepatotoxcicity," Biol Pharm Bull 12 (2002): 1645–1646.

69. H. Hewitt et al., "Topical use of Papaya in chronic skin ulcer therapy in Jamaica," West Indian Med. J. 49, 1 (2000): 32–33.

70. I. F. Starley et al., "The treatment of paediatric Burns using topical papaya," Burns 25 (1999).

71. R. Giordani et al., "Fungicidal activity of latex sap from Carica papaya and anti-fungal effect of D-(+)-glucosamine on Candida albicans," Mycoses 39, 3–4 (1996): 103–110.

72. L. Tona, K. Kambu, and N. Njimbi, "Anti-amoebic and phytockemical screening of some Congolese medicinal plants," J. Ethnopharmacol 61, 1 (1998): 57–65.

73. C. F. Chen et al., "Protective effects of Carica papaya Linn on the exogenous gastirc ulcer in rats," Am J Chin Med 9, 3 (1981): 205–212.

74. J. A. Osato et al., "Antimicrobial and anti-oxidant activities of unripe papaya," Life Sci. 53, 17 (1993): 1383–1389.

75. O. O. Oyedapo and B. G. Araba, "Stimulation of protein biosynthesis in rat hepatocytes by extracts of Momordica charantia," Phytotherapy Research 15 (2001): 95–98.

76. T. O. Bamidele et al., "The modulatory effect of Momordica charantia on the plasma and intestinal Ca_2+ ATPase in normal and alloxan-induced diabetic rabbits," Nigerian Journal of Pharmaceutical Research 1, 1 (2002): 26.

77. A. U. Ogan, "An oxytocic extractive from a West African cucurbit: studies on West African Medicinal Plants-8," Planta Medica 21, 4 (1972): 431–434.

78. J. A. O. Ojewole and A. A. Elujoba, "Preliminary investigation of the oxytocic action of an aqueous extract of Lagenaria breviflora fruit," International Journal of Crude Drug Research 20, 4 (1982): 157–163.

79. A. A. Elujoba, S. Olagbende, and S. K. Adesina, "Anti-implantation activity of the fruit of Lagenaria breviflora Robert," Journal of Ethnopharmacology 13 (1984): 281–288.

80. Aphrodite T. Choumessi et al., "Cell division," 7, 8 (2012), accessed 1/3/16, http://www.com/content/7/1/8.

81. J. Welihinda et al., "Effect of Momordica charantia on the glucose tolerance in maturity unset diabetes," J. Ethnopharmacol 17, 3 (1986): 277–282.

82. S. Sarkar, M. Pranava, and R. Marita, "Demonstration of the hypoglycaemic action of Momordica charantia in validated animal model of diabetes," Pharmacol Res. 33 (1996): 1–4.

83. T. B. Ng et al., "Insulin-like molecules in Momordica charantia seeds," J. Ethnopharmacol 15 (1986): 107–117.

84. P. Khanna et al., "Extraction of insulin from a plant source," 3rd International Congress on Plant Tissue and Cell Cultures (July 21–26, 1974), Leicester, UK.

CHAPTER 13

The Cellular Mechanisms by Which Inhibitory and Excitatory Effects of Medicinal Plants Are Produced in the Body of Living Organisms

THE SMALLEST UNITS of the body of organisms are called cells. Cells are therefore the "building blocks" of living organisms at which the basic processes and activities that keep the organism alive are carried out. The cells of every organ of the body are slightly modified to fit the function that organ provides for the body. For example, the cells of the ear are modified for receiving, conducting, and interpreting sound waves while the cells of the tongue are modified to carry out reception and interpretation of different types of chemically elicited tastes (salty, sweet, bitter, sour), and the cells of the eye are modified for reception and interpretation of light stimulus and so on.

One thing that is common to cells of all organ systems of the body is that at the surface of each cell is a site, the cell surface receptor at which the sound stimulus, chemical stimulus, light stimulus, or mechanical stimulus interacts with the cell to cause inhibition or excitation of activities, which affect the cell and consequently the organ and the organ system which the cell is the unit of.

It is at this cell surface receptor site that food is assimilated into the body. Body chemical modulators (like vitamins and hormones), enzymes, and coenzymes as well as exogenous substances (like drugs and plant extracts/juices) act to modulate body activities. Both endogenous compounds like hormones and exogenous compounds like drugs and chemical constituent of plant medicinal extracts and juices, attach to cell surface receptors and interact with the body at the cell surface receptors of cells of organs of the body like the heart, the lungs, the liver, the spleen, the kidney, the intestine, the eye, the brain, etc.

Excitable tissues of living organisms (nerves, muscles, and glands) produce a biphasic (contraction and relaxation) response to maintain the normal tone of the tissue or to produce pharmacological and physiological effects in the body also respond with contraction or relaxation or both contraction and relaxation when stimulated by chemical, electrical, light, sound, and other stimuli. An example of the biphasic response of organisms to intrinsic tonal stimulation and electrical field stimulation is shown in figure 1, which shows the response of chick rectum to tonal and electrical field stimulation.

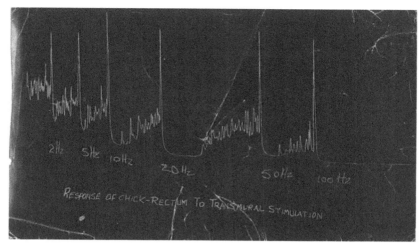

Figure 1. Normal tonic and electrical field stimulation responses of the smooth muscles of the chick rectum. Chick rectum smooth muscles responded to both tonic and electrical field stimulation with 2 hertz, 5 hertz, 10 hertz, 20 hertz, 50 hertz and 100 hertz of electricity with biphasic responses which consisted of a contraction (upward spike) followed immediately by a relaxation (downward vertical stroke or dip)[5].

How Medicinal Plant Extracts Produce Inhibitory Effects at Cell Surface Receptors of the Body of Host Organisms

Both papaverine and atropine were assayed on chick rectum smooth muscles in isolated tissue organ bath experiments.

Papaverine

Papaverine is a naturally occurring alkaloid of opium, a Mediterranean plant of the family *Papaveraceae*, which was discovered in 1848 by Georg Merck (1825–1873).[1] Papaverine is obtained from the plant *Paparver somniferum*, which is used in folk medicine as an analgesic and a soporific.[2]

Papaver belongs to the family *Papaveraceae*. The Paperveraceae family contains twenty-six genera and about three hundred species. Some of the Paperveraceae genera are *Romneya*, *Platysstemon*, *Eschscholtzia*, *Sanguinaria*, *Chelidonium*, *Bochonia*, *Glaucium*, *Meconopsis*, *Argemone*, and *Papaver*.[3] Plants of the family *Papaveraceae* are usually herbs with solitary showy flowers and their fruit is usually a capsule with numerous seeds. All members of the *Papaveraceae* family contain latex tissue which may be in "vessels" that accompany vascular tissue or in sacs. *Papaveraceae* family is rich in alkaloids such as the opium alkaloids.

The behavior of papaverine (a medicinal plant) in this isolated tissue pharmacological research experiment in which papaverine was assayed on chick rectum is a very appropriate demonstration of how medicinal plant extracts produce their effects on living tissues of the organs of animals or humans.

In the assay of papaverine on chick rectum smooth muscles, papaverine produced a large relaxation or inhibitory response at chick rectum smooth muscles, which are shown in figure 2. An inhibitory response is indicated as the tracing of the response going down below the baseline tracings left by the normal tonal contractions and relaxations of the muscle.

This inhibitory response produced by papaverine inhibited tonal biphasic responses of chick rectum smooth muscles while it lasted. Even after the tissue of chick rectum, smooth muscles seemed to have recovered to a new lower baseline after the inhibitory response produced by papaverine, the remnant inhibitory effect of the administered papaverine greatly reduced the heights of the responses of the tissue to electrical field stimulation of two pulses per second and five pulses per second as seen in figure 2.

Note also that the large inhibitory response produced by papaverine blocked any contractions of chick rectum smooth muscles in response to tonal or external excitatory stimulations while it lasted.

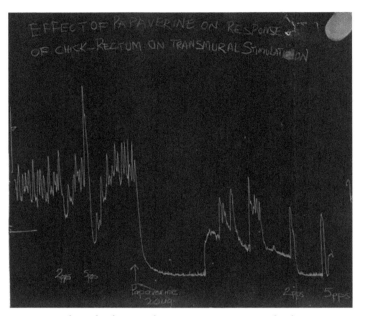

Figure 2. Papaverine produced a large relaxation response at chick rectum smooth muscles which inhibited tonal biphasic response while it lasted and later greatly reduced the heights of the responses of the tissue to electrical stimulation by currents of 2 pps and 5 pps strengths even after the tissue seemed to have recovered to a new lower baseline.[5]

Medicinal plant extracts and their isolates produce inhibitory effects in the body in a similar way as Papaverine did in chick rectum smooth muscles. The extent of the inhibitory effects of a medicinal plant constituent will depend on its structure.

How Medicinal Plant Extracts Produce Excitatory Effects in the Body

Atropine was assayed on chick rectum smooth muscles in the same isolated tissue experiments in which papaverine was assayed. Atropine, also called dl-hyoscyamine, is a belladona alkaloid obtained from the solanaceous plant called the deadly nightshade.

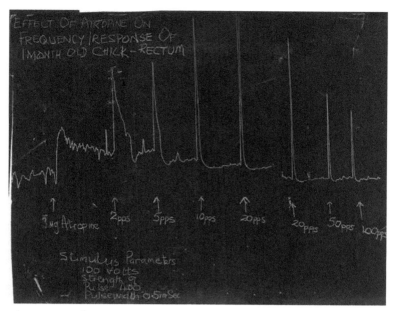

Figure 3. In this tracing, the sustained contraction (excitatory response) produced by atropine (1 µg) coupled to the contraction responses of chick rectum smooth muscles to 2 pps (pulses per second) and 5 pps stimulation, thereby making these two responses to be sustained in comparison to the contractile responses of the same muscles to stimulation by electrical stimuli of 10 pps, 20 pps, 50 pps, and 100 pps stimulation that came after them. Note also that even the remnant powerful contraction produced by atropine continued to be coupled to the responses of the chick rectum smooth muscles to electrical stimuli of 10 pps, 20 pps, 50 pps, and 100 pps as it totally blocked the relaxation phase of the biphasic responses of the tissue to 10 pps, 20 pps, 50 pps, and 100 pps electrical stimulation.[4]

It is this sustained excitatory response of body tissues to atropine that produces the signs and symptoms of atropine poisoning that include difficulty in swallowing; dilated pupils; tachycardia; fever; delirium; stupor; and rash on the face, neck, and upper trunk.[5]

When assayed on chick rectum smooth muscles, atropine elicited a powerful sustained contraction of chick rectum smooth muscles shown in figure 3, which is seen as a spike upward from the level of the normal contractions and relaxations of the muscle that maintain the normal tone of the muscle. The powerful contraction of the smooth muscles of the chick rectum created by atropine lasted for many minutes and created a new higher level of the tonal contractions and relaxations of the tissue (see figure 3).

Note also that this sustained contraction produced by atropine (which is an excitatory response produced by (1 µg) atropine), coupled to both the intrinsic tonal response of chick rectum smooth muscles and to the contraction responses of chick rectum smooth muscles to electrical stimulation, thereby making the tracings of these responses wider as seen in figure 3. Also, contraction response of atropine coupled to contraction responses of the chick rectum smooth muscles to electrical stimulation of 2 pps and 5 pps in figure 3, thereby making these two responses to be sustained in comparison to the contraction responses of the tissue to stimulation of the tissue with the electrical stimulus of 10 pps, 20 pps, 50 pps, and 100 pps. This is how contraction produced by medicinal plant extracts can become sustained in the tissues of the body and can couple to the normal contractions of body cells of humans, animals, or plants to which they are administered.

Note also that during the sustained powerful contraction of the chick rectum smooth muscles by atropine, this contraction inhibited the relaxation of the muscles for as long as this sustained contraction lasted. This is probably what earned the plant the name the "deadly" nightshade. Medicinal plant extracts that produce very powerful sustained contractions or excitations will similarly inhibit relaxation of the tissues and organs in which they have produced such contractions or excitatory responses.

Conclusions

These two examples of how papaverine produced a large, deep relaxation response and atropine produced powerful large sustained contraction at the same cell surface receptors of cells of chick rectum smooth muscles have demonstrated that medicinal plant extracts and their chemical constituents produce inhibitory and excitatory effects at the same cell surface receptors of host organisms. These two examples have also demonstrated that inhibitory and excitatory effects of drugs or medicinal plant extracts, at the same cell surface receptors, antagonize and block each other if their magnitude is greater than that of the opposing effect.

In a similar way inhibitory effects of medicinal extracts that are of large and deep magnitude antagonize or block excitatory effects of normal muscle tone or other administered substances, while they last in the body. Inhibitory effects of medicinal plant extracts similarly block excitatory effects on the body produced by body deranging agents like infective agents, chemical agents, or excitatory effects produced by health disorders.

The opposite of what we have seen with relaxation response happens with contraction response to endogenous or exogenous substances. The effects of the excitatory effects produced by administered drugs or medicinal plant extracts, inhibit or excite the release or action of endogenous substances like hormones, saliva; tear; mucous, bile; or the response to other administered drugs or medicinal plant extracts.

References

1. Wikipedia, "Papaverine," last modified September 1, 2015, https://en.wikipedia.org/w/index.php?tittle=Papaverine&o1did= 6700 6859.
2. PubChem, "Structure of Atropine," https://pubchem.ncbi.nlm.nih.gov/compound/atropine#section=3D-Conformer.
3. Ibid.
4. Utoh-Nedosa Uchechukwu Anastasia (2013) Evidence that Adrenergic; Muscarinic; Histaminic; Anti-malarial drugs; Opioid; NSAID, Nicotinic; Vasodilator drugs; Rauwolfian alkaloid and Adenosine Receptors are Parts or Whole of the Serotonin Receptor: chick rectum studies, Presented in Track 3 (Clinical Pharmacy and its Key Role in Treatment), International Summit on Clinical Pharmacy and Dispensing, Nov. 18–20, Hilton San Antonio Airport Hotel, Texas, U. S. A.
5. The Free Dictionary, "Atropine poisoning/definition of atropine poisoning," https://medical-dictionary.thefreedictionary.com/atropine+poisoning accessed 10/5/18.

CHAPTER 14

The Characteristics of Chemical Constituents of Medicinal Plant Extracts Govern Whether the Extracts Will Produce Largely Excitatory or Inhibitory Effects in the Body

MEDICINAL PLANT EXTRACTS usually contain several chemical constituents. Some of these chemical constituents produce inhibitory effects in the body of an organism to which the constituent is administered while others produce excitatory effects.

Since many crude plant extracts contain mixtures of inhibition-producing and excitation-producing constituents, the inhibitory or excitatory effect produced by a crude plant extract reflects the preponderance of inhibition or excitation it produced after the summation of effects produced by the inhibition-producing and the excitation-producing constituents of the crude extract. Thus, if the constituents that produce inhibitory effects predominate in an extract, that extract will produce predominantly inhibitory effects and vice versa.

The excitatory or inhibitory effects produced by medicinal plant extracts can vary in degrees. An extract can produce mildly stimulant or strongly stimulant effects. Similarly, an extract can produce mild, moderate, or strong inhibition of some body activity or many body activities.

The characteristics displayed by the extracts of seven medicinal plants will be presented below to enable us to learn from the plants themselves whether we can off-handedly predict the effect their extract will produce in the body from a knowledge of their general nature. The seven medicinal plants are the following:

1. Black pepper (*Piper guineense*, family Piperaceae)
2. Cinnamon (*Cinnamomum zeylanicum*, family Lauraceae)
3. Ginger rhizome (*Zingiber officinal*, family Zingiberaceae)
4. Grains of paradise (family Zingiberaceae)
5. *Nauclea* (*Nauclea latifolia*, family Rubiaceae)
6. *Fagara* (*Xanthoxylum xanthoxyloides*, family Rutaceae)
7. Guava leaf (leaf of *Psidum guajava*, family Myrtaceae)

If I were asked to suggest the predominant effect the extract of each of these medicinal plants would produce in the body, I would, from a knowledge of the general nature of these medicinal plants and (and their common usage), suggest that black pepper, ginger, and grains of paradise would produce excitatory effects in the body because they are acidic or peppery in nature. I would also say that extracts of cinnamon and guava leaf will produce mild excitatory effects in the body because they are mildly acidic. For the extracts of *Nauclea* and *Fagara*, I would predict that they would produce inhibitory effects in the body because Nigerians use Fagara stem as a bitter chewing stick for cleaning teeth and Nigerian goats feed on Nauclea leaves as a bitter vegetable fodder.

The constituents and medicinal effects of the extracts of each of these plants are listed in table 1. The table allows for a comparison of the effects of each medicinal plant with those of other plants. From the table also, one can easily determine whether my prediction of the effect of the extracts of each of these plants in the body, is correct.

Table 1. A comparison of the chemical constituents and known medicinal effects[1] of the herbal extracts of black pepper, cinnamon, ginger rhizome, grains of paradise, *Nauclea* plant, *Fagara*, and guava leaf to determine whether each of these plants produces predominantly excitatory or inhibitory effects in the body.

Name of Medicinal Plant	Chemical Constituents	Medicinal Effects of Plant Extracts
1. Black pepper (*Piper guineense* Schum and Thonn, family Piperaceae)	Volatile oils, alkaloids, piperine, dihydropiperine, wisanine, dihydrowisanine, sesamin, aschantin, resin and lignans-dihydrochubebin	Antifungal, antimicrobial (i.e., against *Candida*, *Klebsiella*, and *Mycobacterium*), antiviral, insect-repellant, insecticidal, housefly-toxicant, anticonvulsant, oxytocic, oestrogenic, tranquilizing, and sedative effects
2. Cinnamon (*Cinnamomum zeylanicum* Nees, family Lauraceae)	Volatile oils (eugenol, cinnamaldehyde, and phellandrene), coumarins, diterpenoids, triterpenoids, alkaloids, gum, phlobatannins, anthocyanins, mucilage, and calcium oxalate	Antifungal, antibacterial, antiseptic, antihelminthic, astringent, uterine-stimulant, lipolytic, spasmolytic, bittering, digestive-tonic, and appetizing effects
3. Ginger rhizome (*Zingiber officinale* Roscoe, family Zingiberaceae)	Volatile oil (oleoresins), gingerols, monoterpenes (8-phellandrene, (+)-camphene, cineole, borneol, and citral), sesquiterpenes (zingiberene and bisabolene), phosphatidic acid, vitamin C, vitamin B group (riboflavin, niacin, and thiamine), folic acid, mucilage, lecithins, and reducing sugars	Relief of cough, nausea and vomiting of pregnancy, flatulence, indigestion, bloating, lack of appetite, exhaustion, poor circulation, joint pains, boils, chilblains, and hemorrhoids
4. Grains of paradise (*Aframomum melegueta* K. Schum, family Zingiberaceae)	Volatile oils (gingerol, paradol, and shogaol) and oleoresins	Antifungal, antimicrobial, antidiarrheal, antihelminthic, antirheumatic, hemostatic, aromatic stimulant, galactagogue, and purgative effects

5. *Nauclea* (*Nauclea latifolia* Sm, family Rubiaceae)	Indoloquinolizidines (naucletine, nauclefidine, etc.), bitter principles, glycoalkaloids, tannins, resins, and reducing sugars	Antibacterial, antimalarial, antidysentery, antipyretic, diuretic, antihemorrhoids, tonic, and cytotoxic effects
6. *Fagara* (*Xanthoxylum xanthoxyloides* [Lam] Waterm, family Rutaceae)	Essential oils, flavonoids, saponins, alkaloids (fagaramide, fagaridine, fagaronine, berberine, skimmianine, chelerythrine, canthin-6-one, etc.), benzoic acid derivatives (*p*-hydroxybenzoic acid, 2-hydoxymethylbenzoic acid, and vanillic acid), and tannins	Relief/inhibition of fevers, fibrositis, postpartum lower abdominal pain, arterial hypertension, peripheral circulatory insufficiency, edema, chronic rheumatic conditions, impotence, sickle-cell anemia, purulent conjunctivitis, toothache, syphilis of the throat, whooping cough, and wound-healing effects
7. Guava leaf (leaf of *Psidum guajava*, Linn, family Myrtaceae)	Volatile oils (sesquiterpenes, flavonoids [quercetin]), carotenoids, saponins and sapogenins, fiber and fatty acids, starch, vitamin A, vitamin B group (thiamin, nicotinic acid, and niacin), vitamin C, and reducing sugars	Antioxidant, broad-spectrum antimicrobial, vermifuge, antiseptic, antimutagenic, antispasmodic, astringent, analgesic, cardio-protective, antidiarrheal, central-nervous-system-depressant, cough-suppressant, hypoglycemic, and hypotensive effects

The Predominant Effect Produced by Herbal Extracts of Black Pepper, Cinnamon, Ginger Rhizome, Grains of Paradise, *Nauclea* Plant, *Fagara*, and Guava Leaf

The Predominant Effect Produced by Herbal Extracts of Black Pepper

The effects produced by herbal extracts of black pepper include antifungal, antimicrobial (i.e., against *Candida*, *Klebsiella*, and *Mycobacterium*), antiviral, insect-repellant, insecticidal, housefly-toxicant, anticonvulsant, oxytocic, estrogenic, tranquilizing, and sedative effects.[2, 3, 4, 5, 6, 7, 8, 9] Out of these eleven effects listed here, only the oxytocic effect is of an excitatory nature. The ten other effects produced by black pepper (*Piper guineense*) are inhibitory effects. So my prediction that black pepper is acidic and so will produce excitatory effects in the body is wrong because as we have seen here, 91% of the effects produced in the body by black pepper extracts are inhibitory effects.

The Predominant Effect Produced by Herbal Extracts of Cinnamon

The effects produced by herbal extracts of cinnamon include antifungal, antibacterial, antiseptic, antihelminthic, astringent, uterine-stimulant, lipolytic, spasmolytic, bittering, digestive, tonic, and appetizer properties[10, 11, 12, 13, 14, 15, 16, 17].

Out of these eleven effects listed here, only the uterine-stimulant effect is excitatory. The ten other effects produced by cinnamon (*Cinnamonum zeylanicum*) are inhibitory effects. So my prediction that cinnamon is mildly acidic and so will produce mild excitatory effects in the body is correct because as we have seen here, only one of the eleven effects produced in the body by cinnamon extracts is an excitatory effect, which means that 91% of its effects are inhibitory effects. To produce moderate excitatory effects, at least 30%–35% of its effects should be excitatory effects.

The Predominant Effect Produced by Herbal Extracts of Ginger Rhizome

The effects produced by herbal extracts of ginger rhizome (*Zingiber officinale*) include relief of cough, nausea and vomiting of pregnancy, flatulence, indigestion, bloating, lack of appetite, exhaustion, poor circulation, joint pains, boils, chilblains, and hemorrhoids.[18], [19]–33

Out of these thirteen effects listed here, only relief of exhaustion is mildly excitatory. The twelve other effects produced by ginger rhizome are inhibitory effects. So my prediction that ginger rhizome is acidic and so will produce excitatory effects in the body is wrong because as we have seen here, 92% of the effects produced in the body by ginger-stem extracts are inhibitory effects.

The Predominant Effect Produced by Herbal Extracts of Grains of Paradise

The effects produced by herbal extracts of grains of paradise (*Aframomum melegueta*, family Zingiberaceae) include antifungal, antimicrobial, antidiarrheal, antihelminthic, antirheumatic, hemostatic, aromatic stimulant, galactagogue, and purgative effects.[2034], [2135], [2236] Out of the nine effects listed here, only the aromatic stimulant effect is excitatory. This means that 89% of the effects produced in the body by seeds of grains of paradise are inhibitory effects, even though the seeds of *Aframomum melegueta* are very hot (very acidic) in the mouth when they are chewed. Here again, my prediction from the acidic nature of *Aframomum melegueta* seeds that extracts of *Aframomum melegueta* will produce excitatory effects in the body was wrong.

That only 11% of the effects produced in the body by grains of paradise are excitatory suggests that only very high and possibly chronic high doses of extracts of *Aframomum melegueta* will produce its excitatory effects in the body.

The Predominant Effect Produced by Herbal Extracts of *Nauclea* Plant

The effects produced by herbal extracts of *Nauclea* plant listed in table 1 include antibacterial, antimalarial, antidysentery, antipyretic, diuretic, antihemorrhoids, tonic, and cytotoxic effects.[2337], [2438]–44 All of these effects of extracts of *Nauclea* are inhibitory effects. This means that extracts of *Nauclea* (*Nauclea latifolia*) produce 0% excitatory and 100% inhibitory effects in the body. My prediction for these extracts was correct.

The Predominant Effect Produced by Herbal Extracts of *Fagara*

The effects produced by herbal extracts of Fagara (*Xanthoxylum xanthoxyloides*) include relief/inhibition of fevers fibrositis, postpartum lower abdominal pain, arterial hypertension, peripheral circulatory insufficiency, edema, chronic rheumatic conditions, impotence, sickle-cell anemia, purulent conjunctivitis, toothache, syphilis of the throat, whooping cough, and wound-healing effects. All the fourteen effects produced in the body by extracts of *Fagara* are inhibitory effects. This also means that 100% of the effects produced in the body by extracts of *Fagara* are inhibitory effects. My initial guess on these extracts was therefore correct.

The Predominant Effect Produced by Herbal Extracts of Guava Leaf

The medicinal effects produced in the body by herbal extracts of guava leaf include antioxidant, broad-spectrum antimicrobial, vermifuge, antiseptic, antimutagenic, antispasmodic, astringent, analgesic, cardio-protective, antidiarrheal, central-nervous-system-depressant, cough-suppressant, hypoglycemic, and hypotensive effects.[2545, 2646–55] Thirteen out of the fourteen effects of guava (*Psidum guajava*) leaf are inhibitory effects. This means that 93% of the effects produced in the body by guava-leaf extracts are inhibitory. Therefore, guava leaf extract will mostly inhibit diseases and health disorders. One effect out of the fourteen effects produced in the body by guava leaf-extracts is the astringent effect, which is really a very mild excitation at the junction between an inhibitory and an excitatory effect.

Thus, although guava leaf produces a mild sour taste in the mouth, 93% of the effects of extracts of guava leaf in the body are inhibitory effects.

Table 2. The percentage of excitatory and inhibitory effects on diseases and health disorders produced by herbal extracts of black pepper, cinnamon, ginger rhizome, grains of paradise, *Nauclea* plant, *Fagara*, and guava leaf.

Name of Medicinal Plant	Percentage of Excitatory Effects Produced in the Body by Plant's Extracts	Percentage of Inhibitory Effects Produced in the Body by Plant's Extracts
Black pepper (*Piper guineense* Schum & Thonn, family Piperaceae)	9%	91%
Cinnamon (*Cinnamomum zeylanicum* Nees, family Lauraceae)	9%	91%
Ginger rhizome (*Zingiber officinale* Roscoe, family Zingiberaceae)	8%	92%
Grains of paradise (*Aframomum melegueta* K. Schum, family Zingiberaceae)	11%	89%
Nauclea (*Nauclea latifolia* Sm, family Rubiaceae)	0%	100%
Fagara (*Xanthoxylum xanthoxyloides* [Lam] Waterm, Family Rutaceae)	0%	100%
Guava leaf (leaf of *Psidum guajava*, Linn, family Myrtaceae)	7%	93%

Discussions

This review of the effects of extracts of black pepper, cinnamon, ginger rhizome, grains of paradise, *Nauclea* plant, *Fagara*, and guava leaf demonstrated that most medicinal plants produce inhibitory effects in the body. As extracts of these seven medicinal plants examined produce 89%–100% inhibitory effects in the body.

Fagara and *Nauclea*, which are largely alkaline in nature, produced 100% inhibitory effects in the body. Guava leaf, which is mildly sour or mildly acidic, produced 93% inhibitory effects in the body. Ginger stem (which is wrongly called ginger root although it has nodes and internodes, which roots don't have) produced 92% inhibitory effects in the body even though its pungent, acidic taste suggested that it would produce only excitatory effects in the body.

Although in taste, black pepper appears to be more acidic than cinnamon. The fact that extracts of black pepper and cinnamon produced the same 91% inhibitory effects in the body suggests that both plants may have the same level of acidity. The level of acidity in ginger lies midway between that of guava leaf and that of cinnamon/black pepper as ginger extracts produced 92% inhibitory effects in the body, which lies between the 93% inhibitory effects produced by guava leaf extracts and the 91% inhibitory effects produced by black pepper or cinnamon.

Extracts of seeds of grains of paradise seem to be the "hottest" or most acidic of the extracts of the seven medicinal plants examined and were expected to produce 100% excitatory effects in the body. However, the extracts of grains of paradise only managed to produce 11% excitatory effects in the body. The 11% excitatory effects produced by grains of paradise was still the highest percentage of excitatory effects produced by any of the extracts of the seven medicinal plants examined as black pepper/cinnamon, ginger, and guava leaf extracts produced 9%, 8%, and 7% excitatory effects in the body, respectively. Thus, the percentage of excitatory effects exhibited by the medicinal plants increased with the increase in acidity of the plant extract, which was a directly proportional relationship. The reverse was also true of the exhibition of inhibitory effects in the body by the extracts of the seven medicinal plants. The percentage of the inhibitory effects produced in the body by the extracts of the seven plants was directly proportional to the alkaline nature of the plant materials employed, with *Fagara* and *Nauclea* which were the most alkaline substances used in this study, producing 100% inhibitory in the body and no excitatory effects.

Acidity and alkalinity of a plant extract is a characteristic of the molecules of the chemical constituents of the extract. This means that whether a medicinal plant extract will produce largely inhibitory or excitatory effects in the body into which the extract has been taken (administered) is determined by the percentage of the molecules of the medicinally active constituents of the extract that have reactive sites, which will stimulate excitatory or inhibitory responses at the cell surface receptors of tissues of the body of the recipient of the extract.

Conclusion

This review of the effects of the extracts of these seven medicinal plants showed that normal doses of alkaline and also moderately acidic medicinal plants produce largely inhibitory and few excitatory effects in the body. It also demonstrated that the body has very good physiological mechanisms that inhibit moderately acidic medicinal extracts from exacting a high percentage of excitatory effects in the body. The study also demonstrated that extracts of largely alkaline medicinal plant materials produce predominantly inhibitory effects in the body of animals, fellow plants and humans.

References

1. STEPRI (Science and Technology Policy Research Institute), Ghana Herbal Pharmacopoeia (Accra, Ghana: CSIR [Council for Scientific and Industrial Research], 2007).

2. Ibid.

3. A. N. Ngono et al., "Antifungal activity of Piper guineense of Cameroon," Fitoterapia 74, 5 (2003): 464–468.

4. F. V. Udoh, "Uterine muscle reactivity to repeated administration and phytochemistry of the leaf and seed extracts of Piper guineense," Phytother Res. 13, 1 (1999): 55–58.

5. F. V. Udoh, T. Y. Lot, and V. B. Braide, "Effects of Extracts of seed and leaf of Piper guineense on skeletal muscle in rat and frog," Phytother Res. 13, 2 (1999): 106–110.

6. J. I. Olaifa and W. O. Erhun, "Laboratory evaluation of Piper guineense for the protection of cowpea against Callosobrocus maculatus," Insect Science and Its Applications 9, 1 (1988): 55–59.

7. M. Masakazu et al., "Structure, Chemistry and Actions of the Piperaceae amides, new insecticidal constituents isolated from the pepper plant," in Natural Products for Innovative Pest Control, 9th ed., W. S. Bowers and D. L. Whitehead (Oxford Pergamon Press, 1983), 369–382.

8. E. Ayitey-Smith and I. Mensah, "A primary pharmacological study of wisanine, a piperine-type alkaloid from the roots of Piper guineense," West African Journal of Pharmacol and Drug Research 4 (1977): 7–8.

9. R. B. Ashorobi and O. S. Akintoye, "Non-sedating anti-convulsant activity of Piper guineense in mice," Nigerian Quarterly Journal of Hospital Medicine 9, 3 (1999): 231–233.

10. STEPRI (Science and Technology Policy Research Institute), Ghana Herbal Pharmacopoeia (Accra, Ghana: CSIR [Council for Scientific and Industrial Research], 2007).

11. S. Azumi, A. Tanimura, and K. Tanamoto, "A novel inhibitor of bacterial endotoxin derived from cinnamon bark," Biochem Biophys Res Commun 234 (1977): 505–510.

12. J. M. Quale et al., "In vitro activity of Cinnamomum zeylanicum against azole-resistant and sensitive Candida species and a pilot study of cinnamon for oral candidiasis," Am J Clin Med 24, 2 (1996): 103–109.

13. Mancini-Filho et al., "Antioxidant activity of cinnamon, (Cinnamomum zeylanicum)," Breyne, BollChim Farm 137, 11 (1998): 443–447.

14. G. K. Jayaprakasha, M. R. L. Jagan, and K. K. Sakariya, "Volatile constituents from Cinnamomum zeylanicum fruit stalks and their antioxidant activities," J. Agric FoodChem 5, 15 (2003): 4344–4348.

15. H. Nagai et al., "Immunopharmacological studies of the aqueous extract of Cinnamomum cassia (CCAq), 1. Anti-allergic action," Jpn J. Pharmacol 32 (1982): 81322.

16. T. Akira, S. Tanaka, and M. Tabata, "Pharmacological studies on the anti-ulcerogenic activity of Chinese cinnamon," Planta Med 6 (1986): 440–443.

17. L. F. Berrio, M. M. Polansky, and R. A. Anderson, "Insulin Activity-stimulatory effects of cinnamon and brewer's yeast as influenced by albumin," Horm Res 37 (1992): 225–229.

18. STEPRI (Science and Technology Policy Research Institute), Ghana Herbal Pharmacopoeia (Accra, Ghana: CSIR [Council for Scientific and Industrial Research], 2007).

19. J. Backon, "Ginger: inhibition of thromboxane synthetase and stimulation of prostacyclin: relevance for medicine and psychiatry," Med Hypotheses 20 (1986): 271–278.

20. F. Kuchi, S. Iwakami, and M. Shibuya, "Inhibition of prostaglandin and leukotriene biosynthesis by gingerols and diarylheptanoids," Chem. Pharm Bull (Tokyo) 40 (1992): 387–391.

21. H. Bliddal, A. Rosetzsky, and P. Schlichting, "A randomised, placebo-controlled, cross-over study of ginger extracts and ibuprofen in osteoarthritis," Osteoarthritis Cartilage 8 (2000): 912.

22. J. C. Pace, "Oral ingestion of encapsulated ginger and reported self-care actions for the relief of chemotherapy-associated nausea and vomiting," Diss Abstr. Int. 47 (1987): 3297-B.

23. M. E. Bone, D. J. Wilkinson, and J. R. Young, "Ginger root—a new antiemetic. The effect of ginger root on post-operative nausea and vomiting after major gynaecological surgery," Anaesthesia 45 (1990): 669–671.

24. S. Philips, R. Ruggier, and S. E. Hutchinson, "Zingiber officinale (Ginger)—an anti-emetic for day case surgery," Anaesthesia 48 (1993): 715–717.

25. S. S. Sharma et al., "Anti-emetic efficacy of ginger (Zingiber officinale), against cisplatin-induced emesis in dogs," J. Ethnopharmacol 57, 2 (1997): 93–96.

26. S. S. Sharma and Y. K. Gupta, "Reversal of cisplatin-induced delay in gastric emptying in rats by ginger (Zingiber officinale)," J. Ethnopharmacol 62 (1998): 49–55.

27. D. Riebenfeld and L. Borzone, "Randomised double-blind study comparing ginger (Zintona), and dimenhydrinate in motion sickness," HealthNotes Rev. 6 (1999): 98–101.

28. S. L. Vishwakarma et al., "Anxiolytic and anti-emetic activity of Zingiber officinale," Phytother Res. 16, 7 (2000): 621–626.

29. T. Vutyavanich, T. Kraisarin, and R. Ruangsri, "Ginger for nausea and vomiting in pregnancy: randomised, double-masked, placebo-controlled trial," Obstet. Gynecol. 97 (2001): 577–582.

30. H. C. Lien, W. M. Sun, and Y. H. Chen, "Effects of ginger on motion sickness and gastric slow-wave dysrhythmias induced by circular vection," Am J Physil Gastrointest Liver Physiol. 284 (2003): 481–489.

31. M. Blumenthal, "Ginger as an anti-emetic during pregnancy," Altern Ther Health Med. 9 (2003): 19–21.

32. K. C. Srivastava, "Isolation and effects of some ginger components of platelet aggregation and eicosanoid biosynthesis," Prostaglandins Leukot. Med. 25 (1986): 187–198.

33. K. C. Srivastava, "Effect of onions and ginger consumption on platelet thromboxane production in humans," Prostaglandins Leukot. Essent. Fatty Acids 35 (1989): 183–185.

20. 34. STEPRI (Science and Technology Policy Research Institute), Ghana Herbal Pharmacopoeia (Accra, Ghana: CSIR [Council for Scientific and Industrial Research], 2007).

21. 35. K. C. Srivastava and T. Mustafa, "Ginger, Zingiber officinale in rheumatism and musculoskeletal disorders," Med. Hypotheses 39 (1992): 342–348.

22. 36. P. Kamtchouing, G. Y. Mbongue, and T. Dimo, "Effects of Aframomum melegueta and Piper guineense on sexual behaviour of male rats," Behav. Pharmacol 13, 3 (2002): 243–247.

23. 37. STEPRI (Science and Technology Policy Research Institute), Ghana Herbal Pharmacopoeia (Accra, Ghana: CSIR [Council for Scientific and Industrial Research], 2007).

24. 38. S. Umukoro and R. B. Ashorobi, "Pharmacological evaluation of the anti-diarrhoeal activity of Aframomum melegueta seed extract," West Afr. J. Pharmacol. Drug Res. 19, 1 and 2 (2003): 51–54.

39. A. Gidado, D. A. Ameh, and S. E. Atawodi, "Effect of Nauclea latifolia leaves' aqueous extract on blood glucose levels of normal and alloxan-induced diabetic rats," African J. Biotech. 4, 1 (2005): 91–93.

40. P. A. Onyeyili et al., "Anti-helminthic activity of crude aqueous extract of Nauclea latifolia stem bark against ovine nematodes," Fitoterapia 72, 1 (2001): 12–22.

41. S. Amos et al., "Neuropharmacological effects of aqueous extract of Nauclea latifolia root bark in rats and mice," J. Ethnopharmacol 10, 97 (2005): 53–57.

42. M. I. Akpanabiatu et al., "Influence of Nauclea latifolia leaf extracts on some hepatic enzymes of rats fed on coconut oil and non-coconut oil meals," Pharmaceutical Biology (formerly International Journal of Pharmacognosy) 43, 2 (2005): 153–157.

43. I. I. Madubunyi, "Anti-hepatotoxic and Trypanosomacidal Activities of the ethanolic extract of Nauclea latifolia root bark," J Herbs Spices Med. Plants 3, 2 (1995): 23–53.

44. Y. Deeni and Hussain, "Screening for antimicrobial activity and for alkaloids of Nauclea latifolia," J Ethnopharmacol 35 (1991): 9196.

25. 45. STEPRI (Science and Technology Policy Research Institute), Ghana Herbal Pharmacopoeia (Accra, Ghana: CSIR [Council for Scientific and Industrial Research], 2007).

26. 46. O. A. Osoba, S. A. Adesanya, and M. A. Durosimi, "Effect of Zanthoxylum xanthoxyloides and some substituted benzoic acids on glucose-6-phosphate and 6-phosphogluconate dehydrogenases in Hbss red blood cells," J. Ethnopharmacol 27, 1–2 (1989): 177–183

47. P. Jaiarj, "Anti-cough and antimicrobial activities of Psidium guajava Linn leaf extract," J. Ethnopharmacol. 67, 2 (1999): 203–212.

48. X. Lozoya, "Intestinal anti-spasmodic effect of a phytodrug of Psidium guajava folia in the treatment of acute diarrhoeic disease," J. Ethnopharmacol. 83, 1–2 (2002): 19–24.

49. L. Wei et al., "Clinical study on treatment of Infantile rotaviral enteritis with Psidium guajava," Zhong guo Zhong Xi Yi Jie He Za Zhi 20, 12 (2000): 893–895.

50. S. Begum et. al., "Triterpenoids from the leaves of Psidium guajava," Phytchem 61, 4 (2002): 399–403.

51. H. Arima and G. Danno, "Isolation of antimicrobial compounds from guava (Psidium guajava L), and their structural elucidation," Biosci. Biotecnol. Biochem. 66, 8 (2002): 1727–1730.

52. A. Jimenez-Escrig, "Guava fruit (Psidium guajava L) as a new source of antioxidant dietary fiber," J. Agric. Food Chem 49, 11 (2001): 5489–5493.

53. R. B. Singh, "Effects of guava intake on serum total and high-density lipoprotein cholesterol levels and on systemic blood pressure," Am. J. Cardiol. 70, 15 (1992): 1287–1291.

54. J. T. Cheng et. al., "Hypoglycaemic effect of guava juice in mice and human subjects," Am J. Clin. Med. 11, 1–4 (1983): 74–76.

55. I. S. Grover and S. Bala, "Studies on anti-mutagenic effects of guava (Psidium guajava) in Salmonella typhimurium," Mutat. Res. 300, 1 (1993): 1–3.

ABOUT THE AUTHOR

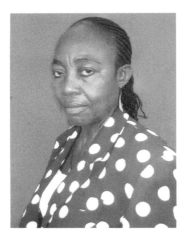

DR. UCHECHUKWU ANASTASIA Utoh-Nedosa has a Bachelor of Science Degree in Pharmacology of the University of Ibadan, Ibadan, Nigeria. She has both a Master's Degree in Health Education and a Doctoral Degree in International and Development Education of the University of Pittsburgh, Pittsburgh, Pennsylvania, United States. She also has a Master of Science Degree in Pharmacology and Toxicology of the University of Nigeria, Nsukka, Enugu State, Nigeria.

As a faculty member, Dr. Uchechukwu Utoh-Nedosa lectured in health education at the Institute of Education of Ahmadu Bello University, Zaria, Kaduna State, Nigeria, and worked as a graduate assistant in the Department of Pharmacology of Faculty of Pharmaceutical Sciences of the same university. She also engaged in teaching and research as a faculty member in the Department of Pharmacology and Toxicology of the Faculty of Pharmaceutical Sciences of Nnamdi Azikiwe University, Awka, Anambra State, Nigeria.

Her hobbies are team sports; organic farming; and educating people to eat health-promoting foods, live healthy lifestyles, and value one another.

CPSIA information can be obtained
at www.ICGtesting.com
Printed in the USA
LVHW071752170222
R17170100001B/R171701PG710938LVX00001B/1